D0552759

Anyone who wants to know about the size of the cancer problem and the scope for prevention should read this book.

We see it as part of a campaign that will lead to a reduction in a significant proportion of cancer that is caused by chemicals in the work place, in the home and in the environment.

The book stands both as a memorial to workers who have died unnecessarily from occupational cancer, and as a guide to further preventative action.

David Basnett General Secretary
General Municipal, Boilermakers' and Allied Trades' Union
(GMBATU)

GATESHEAD COLLEGE
LEARNING CENTRES
16017039
616
.994
DO.Y

The Politics of Health

Editor: Lesley Doyal

This series on the politics of health is concerned with social and environmental causes of ill-health both in Britain and in the third world. It looks at the growing critique of contemporary medical practice as well as the possibility of socialist and feminist alternatives for the creation of a healthy society.

Lesley Doyal

Ken Green, Alan Irwin, Doogie Russell,
Fred Steward, Robin Williams, Dave Gee and

Samuel S. Epstein

Cancer in Britain

The politics of prevention

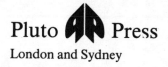

Pluto Press

London and Sydney

First published in 1983 by Pluto Press Limited,
The Works, 105a Torriano Avenue, London NW5 2RX
and Pluto Press Australia Limited, PO Box 199, Leichhardt
New South Wales 2040, Australia

Copyright © Lesley Doyal, Samuel S. Epstein, Dave Gee, Ken Green,
Alan Irwin, Doogie Russell, Fred Steward and Robin Williams 1983

Text designed by Brent Curless
Cover designed by Michael Mayhew

Typeset and printed in Great Britain by Photobooks (Bristol) Ltd
Bound by W. H. Ware and Sons Limited, Tweed Road, Clevedon, Avon

British Library Cataloguing in Publication Data
Cancer in Britain.
  1. Cancer – Prevention – Great Britain
  I. Doyal, Lesley   II. Epstein, Samuel S.
  616.99'405   RC268

ISBN 0-86104-394-4

616.994

B 27204

GATESHEAD
TECHNICAL
COLLEGE
LIBRARY

Contents

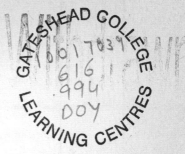

GATESHEAD COLLEGE
00170399
616.
.994
DOY
LEARNING CENTRES

A note on the history of the book

The first edition of *The Politics of Cancer* by Samuel S. Epstein was published as a hardback (Sierra Club Books) in 1978 and an expanded paperback version (Anchor /Doubleday Press) appeared in 1979. It made an immediate impact and played a critical role in the debate about the social and economic determinants of cancer and of cancer prevention in the United States and elsewhere. In 1980, Pluto Press decided to publish a British version of this work.

This was to have included a major part of the original American paperback edition. Several new chapters were added to describe the cancer problem in Britain and explain the workings of the regulatory process. Further British material was also added to illustrate the various case studies. This additional work was carried out, in conjunction with Professor Epstein, by a group of British authors, all of whom have considerable experience – both practical and theoretical – of the relations between health, science and society. The completed work was scheduled for publication as *The Politics of Cancer in Britain and America* by Samuel S. Epstein and Lesley Doyal with Ken Green, Alan Irwin, Doogie Russell, Fred Steward and Robin Williams. At this late stage, however, it became apparent that much of the American work was not appropriate for publication in its original form. For these reasons it was decided to make the British material the basis for a book dealing specifically with the cancer problem in Britain. Naturally, given its history, this book is deeply indebted in inspiration, structure and content to Professor Epstein's pioneering work. Indeed, this volume follows the format of *The Politics of Cancer* closely and the two can most usefully be read in conjunction. The process of preparing the material for publication took the best part of another year and involved detailed collaborative work on the part of all authors. As a result, the book is now entitled *Cancer in Britain: The Politics of Prevention* and the new ascription of authorship reflects this history.

Acknowledgements

The authors would like to thank Mick Carpenter for help with an early draft of chapter two, Dave Eva for help with the case study on pesticides, Sheila McKechnie for help with the sections on the regulatory process and on work-place hazards and Chris Kaufman for help on the 2,4,5-T case study. John Matthews's unstinting help at short notice on the regulation section and on several case studies was especially welcome. This book caused more agonies than most in its gestation and many people are owed thanks for their support and encouragement. Len Doyal and Richard Kuper in particular made it possible to go on when it sometimes seemed the process would never end! Finally, we thank Freddi Cooke, Wendy Millmott, Pat Clarke and Susan Pritchard for typing a difficult manuscript with such efficiency and tolerance.

List of abbreviations

ABPI	Association of the British Pharmaceutical Industry
ACA	Advisory Committee on Asbestos (UK)
ACGIH	American Conference of Government Industrial Hygienists
ACP	Advisory Committee on Pesticides (UK)
ACTS	Advisory Committee on Toxic Substances (UK)
A/D	aldrin and dieldrin
AI	Alkali Inspectorate (UK)
AN	Acrylonitrile
ANHIST	Acrylonitrile Health Impact Study Team (UK)
ASTMS	Association of Scientific, Technical and Managerial Staffs (UK)
BAA	British Agrochemicals Association
BASIS	British Agrochemicals Supply Industry Scheme
BAT	British American Tobacco
BCME	Bischloromethyl ether
BFRMA	British Food Manufacturers Research Association (became BFMIRA, British Food Manufacturers Industrial Research Association)
BIBRA	British Biological Research Association
BOHS	British Occupational Hygiene Society
BP	British Petroleum
BSSRS	British Society for Social Responsibility in Science
CBI	Confederation of British Industry
C/H	chlordane and heptachlor
CIA	Chemical Industries Association (UK)
CISHEC	Chemical Industry Safety and Health Council
COT	Committee on the Toxicity of Chemicals in Food, Consumer Products and the Environment (UK)

CRM Committee on the Review of Medicines (UK)
CSM Committee on the Safety of Medicines (UK)
DBCP Dïbromochloropropane
DES Diethylstilboestrol
DES Department of Education and Science (UK)
DHSS Department of Health and Social Security (UK)
DP Depo-Provera
EEC European Economic Community
EHDs Environmental Health Departments (UK)
EMAS Employment Medical Advisory Service (UK)
EPA Environmental Protection Agency (USA)
FACC Food Additives and Contaminants Committee (UK)
FAFR Fatal Accident Frequency Rate
FDA Food and Drug Administration (USA)
GWMU General and Municipal Workers' Union (UK; became General Municipal, Boilermakers' and Allied Trades' Union)
HRT Hormone Replacement Therapy
HSC Health and Safety Commission (UK)
HSE Health and Safety Executive (UK)
IARC International Agency for Research on Cancer
ICI Imperial Chemical Industries
MAFF Ministry of Agriculture Fisheries and Food (UK)
MASC Manchester Area Safety Committee
MMF Man-made Mineral Fibres
NCI National Cancer Institute
NEDO National Economic Development Organisation
NGA National Graphical Association (UK)
NIEHS National Institute of Environmental Health Sciences (USA)
NIOSH National Institute for Occupational Safety and Health (USA)
NTP National Toxicology Program (USA)
NUAAW National Union of Agricultural and Allied Workers (UK; became Transport and General Workers' Union, Agricultural and Allied Workers' National Trade Group)
OCAW Oil, Chemical and Atomic Workers' Union (USA)

OECD	Organization for Economic Cooperation and Development
OPCS	Office of Population Censuses and Surveys (UK)
OSHA	Occupational Safety and Health Administration (USA)
OTA	Office of Technology Assessment (USA)
PSPS	Pesticides Safety Precaution Scheme (UK)
(P)VC	(poly)vinyl chloride
SMR	Standardised Mortality Ratios
2,4,5-T	2,4,5-Trichlorophenoxyacetic acid
TCDD	2,3,7,8-Tetrachlordibenzo-p-dioxin
TGWU	Transport and General Workers' Union
TLV	Threshold Limit Value
TOSCA	Toxic Substances Control Act (USA)
USDA	Department of Agriculture (USA)
VC	Vinyl chloride
WHO	World Health Organization

1. The politics of cancer

Cancer is increasingly regarded as a preventable disease; accordingly, there has been growing criticism of the curative emphasis that dominates most research. It is generally accepted that most cancers are caused by the way we live and work, and that changes are an essential first step towards prevention. However, there is considerable disagreement about what these changes should be and how they could be brought about. It is this debate about strategies for prevention that provides the major focus for *Cancer in Britain*.

Why has there been a swing towards prevention in the case of cancer in particular? The most immediate reason is probably the sheer size of the problem. The disease now kills one in five of all people dying in Britain. Furthermore, cancer is now the disease that people fear most. Just as tuberculosis appeared to symbolise the wretched conditions of nineteenth-century towns, so cancer has come to be seen as an epidemic that is somehow characteristic of the 'affluent society' of the post-war period.[1] This fear is exacerbated by the fact that western medicine has so far proved remarkably ineffective in helping cancer patients – survival rates for most of the common cancers have improved very little over the past 30 years. Indeed, there is a growing belief that, far from providing a cure, cancer treatment often serves merely to reduce the quality of the patient's remaining life-span.

This growing emphasis on prevention has been reinforced by the recognition that, like the other 'diseases of affluence', cancer is usually both environmental and multi-causal in origin. That is to say, there is not usually a simple relationship between the onset of cancer and exposure to a particular carcinogen. Rather, most cases are related to several different elements in a victim's physical, social and economic environment which interact with his/her own genetic make-up to produce a cancer. The fact that the majority of cancers are largely environmental in origin is evidenced by the marked differences found in cancer rates between different social groups. ('Environmental' is used here in the widest sense, encompassing all those external influences impinging on an individual organism.) This applies to the variations in incidence between different countries but especially to the marked differences between social classes in the *same* country. In Britain, for example, most of the major cancers are more common among semi-skilled and unskilled workers than among their more affluent compatriots (see chapter 2). Lung and stomach cancers in particular show a very marked social class differential of this kind. These class differences are important, not just because they illustrate yet another of the burdens disproportionately borne by the underprivileged in our society, but because they demonstrate that cancer cannot be explained simply in natural or genetic terms. Instead, it has to be understood as one outcome of the material differences that exist between the lives of people in different social groups.

From a public health perspective, the central tasks in any prevention campaign would therefore be the removal or transformation of those aspects of people's lives that render them more likely than others to develop cancer. However, as soon as we move into the formulation of practical strategies for achieving such a goal, political concerns immediately become apparent. Contrary to popular mythology, issues of this kind are never resolved by reference to purely scientific considerations, as we can see if we look at the current debate about cancer prevention in Britain. Two distinct positions are clearly identifiable. Each has its own view about the relative importance of the different causes of cancer, its own recommendations about how the disease could be prevented, and, underlying both of these, its own political philosophy. At the risk of oversimplification, we will call these the 'establishment' and the 'radical' approaches, though there is inevitably some degree of overlap between the two.

If we look first at the 'establishment' approach, it is clear that the most vociferous proponents of this view are industrial interests – the Chemical Industries Association (CIA) in particular. However it is also to be found in many official government publications where the emphasis is on individuals looking after their own health, rather than expecting the state to do it for them. The 'establishment' approach rests on two major assumptions. First, it is argued that industrial products and processes play very little part in causing cancer. Thus, occupational factors are said to cause less than 5 per cent of all cancers and pollution some 2 per cent. Instead, the major causes of cancer are said to be smoking (causing some 30 per cent of all cancers) and diet (about 35 per cent). Additional factors often mentioned are alcohol, food additives, sunshine and 'sexual habits'. According to this view, the most significant causes of cancer are things to which individuals willingly expose themselves, so that social class differences are explained by the assumption that working-class people *voluntarily* lead less healthy lives than their more enlightened fellows. Whether this is because of moral weakness, intellectual inferiority, lack of education or sheer laziness is never made clear. In any case, the main hope for prevention is seen to lie in more health education – in trying to persuade people to 'look after themselves'.

In order to back up their analysis, exponents of the 'establishment' approach tend to draw heavily on the work of Richard Doll and Richard Peto. Doll and Peto are influential cancer epidemiologists; their recent volume *The Causes of Cancer* (1982) has been extremely important in supporting industry's position. It is necessary, therefore, to look carefully at the social implications of their approach and at the uses to which their work has been put. In particular, we need to look at the ways in which their ideas have been used to reinforce the 'victim blaming' approach that has been prominent in recent discussions of ill-health in general and cancer in particular. Of course, the technical arguments used to support the 'establishment' position are always put forward in apparently neutral and value-free terms and Doll and Peto have gone to considerable trouble to assert their own impartiality.[2] However, their ideas have been eagerly seized upon by industry and widely disseminated by the CIA in their attempts to resist further regulation.

The alternative approach to cancer – which we have called the 'radical' view – is taken by trade unions, environmental groups and others concerned to expose the role of industry in the creation of ill-health. According to this view, industrial processes and hazardous chemicals play a far more significant part in the causation of cancer than the 'establishment' position would admit. It recognises the importance of smoking, diet, and other factors individuals could perhaps control, but it places more emphasis on industrial exposures over which the individual has little or no say.

Supporters of this approach have drawn particularly on the work of Samuel Epstein, Professor of Occupational and Environmental Medicine at the University of Illinois and an international authority on the toxic and carcinogenic hazards of chemicals. Epstein supports the 20–40 per cent minimal estimates calculated by a group of American Federal experts for the proportion of cancers that are work-related.[3] He also stresses industrial pollution and the chemicals used in consumer products as significant causes of cancer. Furthermore, he demonstrates that the contribution of smoking, while clearly major (see Appendix 3), has been over-estimated because it is often seen as the *only* cause of a cancer which in fact often has an occupational component. Diet he sees as having little proven relationship with cancer except in the very specific case of deliberate or accidental carcinogenic food additives.

According to this view then, the answer to the cancer problem lies not merely in health education – in the moral persuasion of individuals – but in the identification and regulation of hazardous industrial chemicals, whether in the workplace, in consumer products or in the wider environment. Moreover, there is a clear realisation that this greater control will not be achieved by individuals acting alone, and that neither industry nor government can be left to their own devices on the assumption that they will act in the public interest. Thus, it is assumed that the social and economic changes required for any real progress in cancer prevention can only be achieved through collective political action.

In the same way that the CIA have used the Doll–Peto analysis to bolster their case against further regulation of industry, so trade unions have used the analysis of Epstein (and others) in their fight for better health and safety measures at work. Three unions in particular – the Association of Scientific, Technical and Managerial Staffs (ASTMS), the General and Municipal Workers' Union

(GMWU) and the National Graphical Association (NGA) have all produced their own documents exposing the possible carcinogenic hazards facing their workers.[4] In addition the National Union of Agricultural and Allied Workers (NUAAW) has drawn on this analysis in their campaign against 2,4,5-T (see chapter 6).

In Britain there is, therefore, a continuing debate between what we have called the 'establishment' and the 'radical' positions, with skirmishes ranging from debates in the scientific literature[5] to more overtly political battles of words between the CIA and the unions.[6] These debates have been summarised by Peto and Epstein (see appendices 2 and 3 for an outline).

So who is right? This remains a matter of considerable dispute and certainly more information is required before we can come to definitive conclusions about the relative importance of different causes of cancer. However, there are good reasons for suggesting that the CIA calculation of 4–5 per cent of cancers being work-related is a considerable underestimate. The main problem with figures of this kind is that they are based on a supposedly unaccountable residue of cancers when all the causes of the major life-style cancers are added up. Additionally, they ignore consideration of at least 130 substances recognised as animal carcinogens by the International Agency for Cancer Research (IARC) as well as a growing number of potentially hazardous substances in daily use that have not yet been adequately tested.[7] Furthermore, it is becoming increasingly clear that many of the carcinogens found in the workplace may spread or be discharged into the air and water of local communities and also may be transmitted directly to others – especially the worker's family. Evidence of this has been found among the families of asbestos workers and there is also growing concern that some proportion of cervical cancer may be caused by the male worker exposing his partner to carcinogens during intercourse.[8] Thus figures reflecting only direct (usually male) exposure are inevitably too low. Finally, it is clear that we still know far too little about the environmental pollution caused by industrial production in Britain, so that it is impossible to make an accurate estimate of its effects on the incidence of cancer.

It seems likely then, that the proponents of the 'radical' view are right in claiming that the industrial–occupational causes of cancer are far more significant than industry cares to admit. A campaign for the identification and control of these substances is therefore of paramount importance if avoidable cancers are to be prevented. Indeed, it is worth pointing out that Doll and Peto themselves (if not their corporate supporters) have recognised that even if 'only' about 4 or 5 per cent of cancers (i.e. 6,000–7,000 per year) are work-related then the detection of such hazards should have a greater priority in any programme of cancer research. Once they are identified, it is usually practicable to remove such hazards – or at least to reduce them quite markedly – and, given the multi-causality of most cancers, this would be likely to reduce the incidence not just of known occupational cancers but also of some not usually seen as directly occupational in origin. It is for this reason that our main focus in this book will be on those occupational and environmental causes of cancer that are relatively easy to remove – given the political will to do so.

It is important to emphasise, however, that any cancer prevention campaign that restricted itself to the control of industrial carcinogens would inevitably be limited in its effectiveness. Even if we achieve a greater degree of control over industrial chemicals we would still be left with significant causes of cancer untouched – smoking in particular. While continuing to campaign for the removal of carcinogenic hazards, we also need to treat smoking, unhealthy diets* and possibly other 'life-style' factors as serious problems that necessitate the development of an appropriate political response.

If we take the example of smoking, for instance, we must accept that cigarettes are probably the single most important cause of preventable cancer and that they kill proportionately more semi-skilled and unskilled workers. It is also clear that not only is smoking a major cause of illness among smokers themselves but what is called 'passive smoking' may also pose a serious threat to those around them. It is essential, therefore, that we develop a clearer understanding of why people smoke cigarettes (or eat unhealthy food) and particularly why such activities should be

---

* In particular, with reference to the relation between high fat diet and cardiovascular disease and the intake of fat soluble carcinogens.

class-related. Whilst not ignoring the question of personal responsibility entirely, we do need to challenge the simplistic 'victim-blaming' approach of industry. We need to highlight the activities of the tobacco industry in persuading people to smoke, and to show how conditions at work and at home may push people to seek solace in cigarettes. Thus, a progressive approach to cancer prevention needs to identify both the industrial causes of cancer and also the social and economic pressures that may lead individuals to act in ways that damage their health. It is only on this basis that an effective strategy for the prevention of cancer can be formulated.[9]

2. The cancer problem in Britain

During the twentieth century there has been a dramatic increase in the number of people suffering and dying from cancer in Britain. In 1901, infectious diseases were the major killers – influenza, pneumonia and bronchitis caused 16 per cent of all deaths while dysentery and diarrhoea accounted for another 7 per cent.[1] Tuberculosis alone killed twice as many people as cancer, which was responsible for only 4.5 per cent of all deaths. By contrast, at least 20 per cent of people now alive in Britain can expect to die from cancer, and the so-called 'diseases of affluence' – cancer and heart disease – now account for about 50 per cent of all deaths.[2] In this chapter, we examine the main features of the cancer problem in Britain. We show that a considerable proportion of the cancer burden arises from past exposure to carcinogenic substances in the general environment, at home and at work, and that much of this exposure results from the pursuit of corporate profit in a situation where public controls are weak.

Cancer in Britain: the overall impact

Over 130,000 men and women died of cancer in England and Wales in 1980 and the disease was the cause of about 22 in every 100 deaths. Cancer is a major cause of death among men and women of all ages. It is the most common cause of death for people aged 35–54 and the second most common cause (after heart disease) for those aged 55–74. Moreover, contrary to popular belief, cancer is not only a disease of middle or old age, but is second only to accidents as a cause of death in those aged 5–34 (see figure 2.1).

In 1979 cancer of the lung claimed most male cancer victims (39 per cent), cancers of the intestine (11 per cent) and stomach (9 per

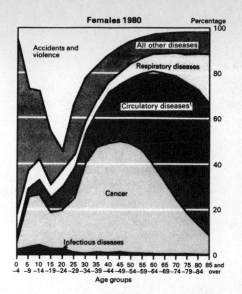

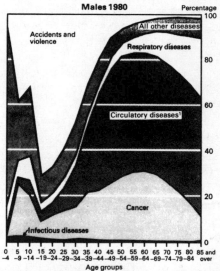

¹ Includes heart attacks and strokes

Figure 2.1 Selected causes of death in the UK, by age and sex, 1980
(source *Social Trends*, no. 13, Central Statistical Office, 1982)

cent) being the other major killing sites (see table 2.1). In the same year, most cancer deaths among women were due to breast cancer (21 per cent), followed by cancers of the intestine (16 per cent), and lung (14 per cent).

Table 2.1 Male and female deaths from cancer in England and Wales, 1979 (source *Mortality Statistics, 1979*, series DH1 no. 8, OPCS, 1982)

Male			Female		
Site	Number of deaths (thousands)	As % of all cancer deaths	Site	Number of deaths (thousands)	As % of all cancer deaths
Lung, bronchus, trachea	26.8	39	Breast	12	21
Intestine, rectum	7.8	11	Intestine, rectum	8.9	16
Stomach	6.5	9	Lung, bronchus, trachea	7.9	14
Prostate	4.8	7	Stomach	4.7	8
Bladder	2.9	4	Ovary	3.7	6
Pancreas	3.0	4	Cervix	2.1	6
Other	18.4	26	Pancreas	2.8	5
			Uterus	3.6	2
			Other	13.0	22
Total	67.7	100		58.7	100

So far we have been talking about the numbers of people who die from cancer (cancer mortality rates) rather than the number who contract it (cancer incidence rates). In the case of an illness which has a high rate of cure, mortality figures of this kind would obviously provide an inaccurate picture of the real extent of the problem. However, in Britain, as in the USA, the 'curability' of most major cancers, particularly of the lung, breast and colon, has improved only slightly over the past three decades.[3] Hence, on an overall basis, and for most major sites, mortality rates closely reflect incidence rates. In the case of lung cancer, for instance, only about 7 patients out of every 100 remain alive 5 years after diagnosis. Even for the more 'curable' breast cancer, just over half of its victims survive 5 years (see table 2.2).

Table 2.2 Number of male and female patients surviving 5 years or more out of every 100 diagnosed with cancer* (source *Cancer Statistics: Survival, 1971–73 Registrations*, series MB1 no. 3, OPCS, 1980)

		Year of diagnosis		
		1959	1964–6	1971–3
Stomach	M	5.5	5.8	7.3
	F	5.7	5.6	7.2
Large intestine	M	23.6	26.2	29.6
	F	23.4	26.3	29.3
Pancreas	M	1.8	1.8	3.78
	F	1.7	2.0	3.12
Lung	M	4.3	6.0	7.8
	F	4.6	5.0	7.0
Breast	M	54.5	51.6	59.5
	F	42.4	51.4	56.8
Cervix	F	39.1	62.0	54.4

* Corrected survival rates.

Evidence of recent increase in cancer rates

Cancer is therefore a major cause of death in Britain and its contribution to the total mortality rate is increasing. There has been a steady rise in crude cancer death rates during this century, and between 1951 and 1975 rates among British males increased by about 1 per cent per year.[4] Cancer death rates among women fell by some 7 per cent between 1943 and 1963; since that period, they have been on the increase and, like male rates, rose by about 1 per cent per year during the 1970s.[5] Obviously the 'epidemic' of lung cancer during the post-war period has been the major factor in this rise, but in men, there have also been increases in deaths from leukaemia and bladder and pancreatic cancers, while in women there has been a marked increase in breast cancer since 1961 and steady increases in cancers of the ovary and pancreas. Rates for stomach and intestinal cancer declined among both sexes between 1951 and 1971, but mortality rates from intestinal cancer are now beginning to rise again among men. In fact, stomach and cervical cancers are the only major cancers to have shown a consistent decline during the post-war period.[6]

It is often suggested that this increase in cancer mortality is merely an artefact of the statistics, reflecting the increasing number of older people in the population. Thus, it is argued, the increase would disappear if we adjusted for these demographic changes. However, when the crude mortality figures are adjusted to take into account the proportion of the population in different age groups, the adjusted death rate from cancer has still risen – though not quite so steeply as the crude death rate.[7] It is clear, therefore, that we are dealing with a real and absolute rather than an apparent and relative increase in cancer deaths.

How are we to explain these real increases in cancer mortality? The most obvious explanation might be that the figures simply reflect improvements in diagnosis – that more cancer deaths are now recognised for what they are and recorded as such. There is no doubt that this has played some part in the increase, but the overall effect is likely to be small, particularly in recent decades. An alternative and widely held assumption is that the increase in the number of people dying from cancer, if not an artefact of the statistics, is nevertheless a 'natural' and inevitable consequence of an ageing population. 'You've got to die of something,' is a comment frequently heard. Thus it is claimed that with the decline in infectious diseases and an overall improvement in standards of living, people live longer and an increase in cancer is unavoidable – that cancer is simply a 'degenerative' disease which is part of the ageing process itself. But there are certain problems with this argument, the most important being that there has been a real rise in cancer rates in *all* age groups, and a theory which attributes cancer only to 'degeneration' cannot account for this excess mortality at all ages. Given this fact, a more plausible explanation is that an individual's chance of contracting cancer *increases* with greater exposure to carcinogenic substances whose production has in general been much increased in recent decades. For most people, the longer they live the greater that exposure is likely to be and the greater is the opportunity for cancers to develop, following exposure earlier in life. This provides an important additional element in explaining the link between cancer and longevity. Viewed in this way, historical trends in cancer incidence point to the role of environmental factors in producing many types of cancer –

an interpretation which is borne out both by comparative evidence of cancer rates in different societies and also, very importantly, by the marked differences that exist in cancer rates for different groups in the *same* society.

Social class differences in cancer rates

In the United States, evidence concerning different cancer rates among blacks and whites has been used to demonstrate the importance of environmental influences.[8] In Britain, we know very little about such racial differences, but the very obvious and dramatic *class* differences in cancer mortality provide powerful evidence of the impact of environmental factors.[9] An examination of standardised mortality ratios (SMRs)[10] shows that there is a marked difference in death rates from cancer among different social classes, so that people belonging to social classes IV and V[11] are considerably more likely to die from cancer *at any age* than their counterparts in social classes I and II (figure 2.2). Moreover, this

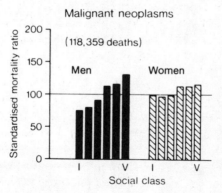

Note This figure includes six bars for five social classes as a result of changes in classification made in 1970. Class III is now divided into two subgroups: IIIN (non-manual skilled occupations) and IIIM (manual skilled occupations).

Figure 2.2 Mortality by social class and cause of death: standardised mortality ratios for men and married women (by husband's occupation) aged 15–64 (source *Occupational Mortality: Registrar General's Decennial Supplement, 1970–72*, series DS no. 1, OPCS, 1978)

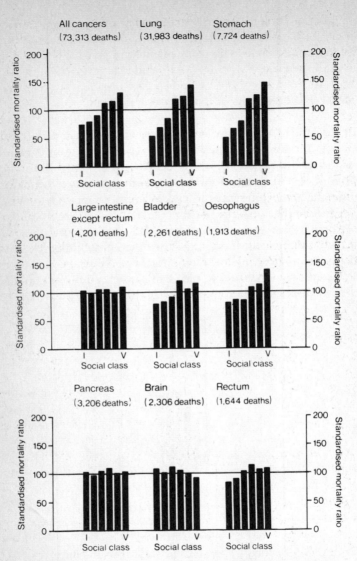

Figure 2.3 Mortality by social class and rank order of major cancer sites in men aged 15–64, 1970–72 (source *Occupational Mortality: Registrar General's Decennial Supplement, 1970–72*, series DS no. 1, OPCS, 1978)

social class gradient is steeper among men than among women – a fact which probably reflects in part their greater exposure to occupational carcinogens.

There are also important variations in the social class gradients for different *types* of cancer (figure 2.3). Social class gradients are most pronounced for lung and stomach cancers which together accounted for more than half the total number of male cancer deaths in 1970–72; the gradient is much shallower for bladder, oesophageal and rectal cancers. Only two forms of cancer – intestinal and pancreatic – are apparently class 'impartial'; while brain cancer has a *negative* social class gradient – i.e. is commonest among those in higher social classes. Thus, among men, cancer at five of the major sites shows a positive social class gradient. Comparable tables are not available for female cancers, and most mortality data classifies married women according to their husbands' occupation, thus obscuring possibly important relationships between women's own work and their cancer risk. However, class differentials are observable in female cancer rates (figure 2.2). Cervical cancer in particular is much more common among women of social class IV and V. However, it is important to note that breast cancer, the commonest cancer among women, is more frequent in *higher* social classes.

It is clear then that there are very significant class differences in overall cancer rates in Britain, as well as in the rates of cancer at different sites. It is unlikely that variations of this kind are merely random, or the result of genetic differences between social groups. We therefore need to examine the lives of people in different social classes in order to assess why men and woman in social class IV and V are more likely to die prematurely of some form of cancer than those who are more affluent.

Most epidemiologists argue that there are two sets of factors primarily responsible for producing these class differences in cancer rates – occupational hazards and the so-called 'life-style' factors.[12] As we have seen in chapter 1, there is still considerable controversy about how many cancers are directly work-related, but we can reasonably assume that a significant, though not precisely quantifiable proportion of cancer can be explained in this way. Leaving these aside, we are then left with the so-called life-style factors commonly used to explain all those cancers that are either unrelated to, or not explicable in terms of occupational exposure alone. Explanations of this kind usually imply that the risks associated with these habits are easily avoidable (compared with the 'unavoidable' ones at work), and result primarily from the moral weakness of the victim. But how useful is 'life-style' as an explanation of class differentials in cancer rates?

As we have seen, the most important problem with this approach is that the way people live is not simply a matter of individual choice – not even in the case of smoking or drinking – but is structured in a multitude of ways by their wider social and economic environment.[13] Moreover the resulting differences in degrees of exposure to carcinogens are not random, but affect those in lower social classes more acutely. People who are most exposed to carcinogens at work are *also* more likely to live in industrially polluted areas, and to smoke heavily; it is this concentration which is largely responsible for such marked class differences in cancer rates. Moreover, it is this very combination of exposures which makes the problem of the relationship between smoking and, say, occupational factors so difficult to disentangle. (In epidemiological terms, smoking and occupation are confounding variables.) Since very few of the studies —other than recent ones—relating smoking to lung cancer have even considered occupation as a relevant variable, there are good grounds for concluding that the relationship between smoking *alone* and lung cancer may well have been overestimated. Indeed such a conclusion is borne out by recent data showing a marked rise in lung cancer rates among non-smokers.[14] 'Life-style' arguments which ignore these facts and offer entirely individualistic explanations are therefore of little value in understanding the real causes of cancer – but of considerable value in covering them up.

We now go on to illustrate these points in more detail by looking at the three most important sources of exposure to carcinogens – the workplace, consumer products and the environment. This discussion will also serve as the background for the case studies provided in chapters 3, 4, 5.

Carcinogens in the workplace

Ever since Percival Pott first pointed out the relationship between scrotal cancer and employment in the chimney-sweeping trade in eighteenth-century Britain, there has been a growing acceptance that certain occupations involve an excess risk of contracting cancer. Indeed, some of these relationships are now so well established that certain cancers are designated as 'prescribed diseases', entitling the victim to possible compensation. Occupational cancers granted this status in Britain include skin cancer caused by exposure to soot, tar and mineral oil (prescribed in 1921); lung cancer caused by exposure to gaseous nickel compounds (1949); bladder cancer caused by aromatic amines in chemical dyestuffs and in rubber production (1953); mesotheliomas caused by exposure to asbestos (1969); adenocarcinoma of the nose caused by exposure to wood dust (1969); angiosarcoma of the liver resulting from exposure to vinyl chloride monomer (1976); and finally, cancer of the nasal cavity contracted in the manufacture and repair of footwear (1979). Thus, for some workers who contract cancer, their disease is recognised as being *possibly* due to occupational exposure and they (or their family) *may* be 'compensated' (see appendix 4 for list of prescribed diseases).

However, only some of the relatively rare cancers are 'prescribed' in this way, and not all workers contracting even these are accepted as victims of occupational exposure. Out of the 4,300 people who died of bladder cancer in Britain in 1976, only five were officially recognised as being entitled to industrial-death benefit.[15] Similarly, we have already seen that even the most minimal estimates recognise that 1–5 per cent of cancers are work related. In the British context, this would give a figure of between 1,200 and 6,000 occupational cancer victims each year. However, in a typical year the Department of Health and Social Security (DHSS) agrees to pay occupational disease-related death benefit to only around a hundred cancer victims.[16] It would seem obvious, then, that even according to the lowest industry estimates, the bulk of occupational cancer still remains uncompensated and even unrecorded. If we look in more detail at the example of asbestos, official statistics acknowledge that 600 people die each year of asbestos-related cancers. Richard Peto

Table 2.3 Occupational cancer in men, 1966–69 (source tables 5G and 5Q in *Occupational Mortality, Registrar General's Decennial Supplement, 1970–72*, series DS no. 1, OPCS, 1978)

Cancer site and sufferer's occupation	Cancer registrations in men aged 15–74	Expected registrations	Excess registrations due to occupational exposure	Excess cancer risk factor*
Lip				
agricultural labourers	68	15	53	5.0
farmers	66	22	34	2.5
construction workers	88	43	45	2.0
labourers	203	116	87	1.8
Salivary gland				
armed forces	34	13	21	2.6
Oesophagus				
agricultural labourers	69	42	27	1.6
textile workers	53	35	18	1.5
Stomach				
miners and quarrymen	1,014	709	305	1.4
glass and ceramic workers	90	65	25	1.4
general metal workers and jewellers	192	136	56	1.4
boiler firemen	138	104	34	1.3
Rectum				
miners and quarrymen	462	362	100	1.3
Liver				
carpenters and joiners	31	20	11	1.3
Pancreas				
coal miners	33	13	20	2.5
tailors	23	12	11	2.0
Nose				
woodworkers	29	15	14	2.0
Larynx				
machine tool operators	80	58	22	1.4
Lung, trachea, bronchus				
ceramic formers	71	48	23	1.4
foundry moulders and coremakers	306	214	92	1.4

Cancer site and sufferer's occupation	Cancer registrations in men aged 15–74	Expected registrations	Excess registrations due to occupational exposure	Excess cancer risk factor*
fettlers and metal dressers	114	81	33	1.4
metal plate workers and riveters	372	281	99	1.3
plumbers, lead burners	491	387	104	1.3
bricklayers and tile setters	845	668	177	1.3
plasterers	238	184	52	1.3
charmen, window cleaners and chimney sweeps	260	198	62	1.3
Skin				
farmworkers, foresters and fishermen	1,148	890	258	1.3
Prostate				
farmworkers, foresters and fishermen	667	496	171	1.3
Bladder				
clothing workers	103	83	20	1.2
rubber workers	42	26	16	1.5
Brain				
farmers and market gardeners	114	78	36	1.5
Hodgkin's disease				
machine tool operators	66	50	16	1.3

* Elevated risk factors do not necessarily imply causal relationships, but should be considered as leads for further epidemiological investigation.

suggests that this figure should be 1,000 (with a twofold uncertainty) while Dave Gee, health and safety officer of the General and Municipal Workers Union, has argued that 2,000 deaths would be more accurate.[17]

But we also need to go beyond the *known* – usually unacknowledged – carcinogenic hazards in the workplace, and consider those that have not, as yet, been investigated. Strong hints of where we might look can be found in the *Registrar General's Decennial Supplement*, as the ASTMS document *The Prevention of Cancer* emphasises (see table 2.3 and appendix 1, p. 158).

The information in table 2.3 is based on the number of cancer registrations from 1966 to 1969 for men in different occupations. These figures are then compared with the number of cancer registrations that would be expected in the general population, making it possible to make some estimate of the number of cancer cases that might be related to particular kinds of industrial exposure. Thus, we find that coal miners, for instance, are two-and-a-half times more likely to get cancer of the pancreas than the rest of the population, while woodworkers are twice as likely to get nasal cancer. With data of this kind, it is obviously difficult to isolate specific causal relationships but as the ASTMS document points out: 'These tables reveal a multitude of links that cannot be ascribed to any substance in particular – but are none the less real and deadly.'[18]

Although we cannot yet explain many of these apparent associations, there are others where the cause – or at least a major contributory factor – is only too obvious. Thus, lung and stomach cancer are strongly associated with work which involves exposure to dusts of various kinds, and exposure to certain metal dusts and fumes is clearly related to an excess risk of lung cancer. Furthermore, it has recently been suggested that we are getting only a very partial view of the carcinogenic effects of such industries by looking at male mortality rates. An examination of the incidence of cervical cancer among married women shows a remarkable association between increased rates of the disease and marriage to men in specific occupations – 'dirty jobs' involving the use of mineral oils, for example.[19]

Carcinogens in consumer products

Cigarette smoking is well recognised as a major cause of lung and other cancers, as well as of other major diseases. There may be synergistic or multiplicative interactions between smoking and certain types of occupational exposure – especially asbestos – in producing an increased risk of lung cancer. Nevertheless, the tobacco industry continues to manufacture and strongly promote cigarettes – a fact which is reflected particularly dramatically in the rising rates of lung cancer among women who are now both smoking more heavily[20] and also becoming increasingly exposed to occupational hazards. Cigarette smoking is, of course, different from most other forms of exposure to carcinogens since it does involve a much greater degree of volition than, say, occupational or environmental exposure. However, as we have already seen, this apparent 'choice' can only be understood in a broader context, since the pressures on people to continue smoking often make it difficult for them to 'choose' to stop – whatever the consequences for their health.

The second potentially carcinogenic consumer product we will be considering is food – a very different sort of commodity from cigarettes. We 'need' food in a way we do not 'need' cigarettes, and yet, like tobacco, some foods may be dangerous to health.[21] Firm evidence has yet to be found, but it seems clear that we need to consider the impact of general dietary composition on cancer incidence. We also need to look particularly carefully at the growing consumption of clearly carcinogenic additives which are either deliberately added to food as colouring agents, preservatives or flavourings, or find their way indirectly into our diet through their use in plastic containers or food wrappings, in cattle feed or as pesticides. Contamination of food with these direct and indirect additives is becoming increasingly common in Britain, yet they are difficult to avoid, since information about their effects is hard to obtain and there are no adequate rules governing the labelling of foods.

Doctors supply us with another important class of consumer product. In Britain, as in the USA, oral contraceptives are now widely used and injectable contraceptives, such as Depo Provera (banned in the USA), appear to be growing in popularity. Hormone-replacement therapy, too, is being prescribed frequently for post-menopausal women.[22] All these drugs have been implicated as causes of some reproductive tract cancers and they do represent a growing – yet largely preventable – cause of cancer among women.

Carcinogens in the general environment

Finally, the general environment is another major potential source of carcinogens. Thus, people may be at risk not only from their jobs and the commodities they consume, but also from the air they must breathe and the water they must drink. The differences between urban and rural cancer rates are very marked in the USA and the same pattern is evident in Britain (see tables 2.4 and 2.5). Thus, it is the industrialised inner-city areas such as Bootle, Islington, Gateshead, Hartlepool and Stoke-on-Trent which show very high rates of lung and stomach cancer.

Table 2.4 County and London boroughs with the greatest excess mortality from cancer of trachea, bronchus, and lung, 1969–73 (source *Area Mortality, 1971*, OPCS, 1980)

Males		Females	
Borough	SMR	Borough	SMR
Bootle	172	Camden	193
Islington	159	Hammersmith	176
Gateshead	152	Westminster	172
Liverpool	152	Southwark	170
Kingston-upon-Hull	152	Lambeth	167
Manchester	151	Islington	162
Salford	151	Salford	158
Newcastle-upon-Tyne	148	Newcastle-upon-Tyne	157
Hammersmith	147	Lewisham	156
Southwark	146	Liverpool	155

It is frequently assumed that these high rates can be explained simply in terms of differences in smoking habits and job patterns, and in the general deprivation found in inner-city areas. However, we do know that the benzpyrene found in soot is a carcinogen, and this gives us good reason to assume that generalised atmospheric pollution also plays a significant part.[23] It is also becoming clear that living close to certain industries and to hazardous waste disposal sites is associated with an increased risk of contracting cancer.[24] So far, we have no cancer maps of the kind that have proved so informative in the USA – indeed, it is only now that British researchers are beginning to look at the relationship between industrial pollution and local patterns of cancer mortality. However, a study carried out in one Scottish town between 1968 and 1974 has revealed a significant excess of deaths from respiratory cancer in those parts of the town exposed to pollution from a steel foundry.[25] This is clearly in line with American findings of increased cancer mortality rates in men and women in communities exposed to industrial pollution – particularly from local petrochemical plants – and we can expect more such data

Table 2.5 Mortality from stomach cancer in selected county boroughs in England and Wales, 1969–73 (source *Area Mortality, 1971,* OPCS, 1980)

	SMR	
	Males	Females
Bootle	163	119
Hartlepool	162	147
Stoke-on-Trent	159	138
Oldham	155	133
Salford	151	134
West Bromwich	148	139
Newport	143	122
Sunderland	138	160
Swansea	133	153
Teesside	132	132
St Helens	127	157
Bolton	125	139
Bury	125	140
Bradford	124	123
Wolverhampton	121	136
Walsall	114	145
Birmingham	113	109
Wigan	111	158
Barrow-in-Furness	104	170

to appear in the near future. Interesting evidence is also emerging from a team in Southampton, about the geographical concentration of occupationally related cancers – an excess of mesothelioma in the dock area of Portsmouth, for instance, and of nasal cancer around High Wycombe where there is a concentration of furniture production (see figure 2.4).[26]

Conclusion

Cancer is a major cause of misery and death in Britain. Moreover, the distribution of hardship falls unevenly on those with least

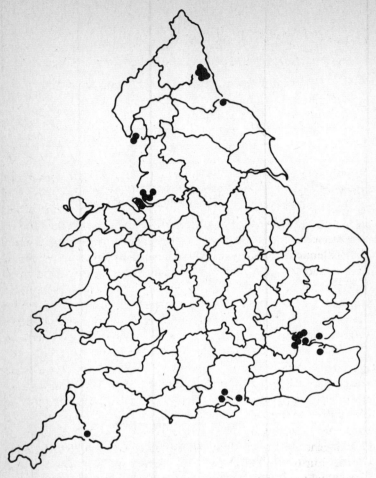

Figure 2.4 'Hot spots' for death from mesothelioma caused by asbestos (source *British Medical Journal*, vol. 284, 1982)

resources. Cancer cannot be explained away as something that just 'happens' to people. Rather, we need to see many cancers as being caused by exposure to carcinogens in the workplace, in consumer products and in the general environment. These cancers are largely preventable – if the real nature of their causes is understood and the fight against them becomes a political priority.

3. How carcinogens are controlled

Introduction

We begin our discussion of the regulatory process in Britain with a brief comparison of policies in the UK and the USA. This is done for several reasons. First, it is useful to consider the outcome of the highly publicised debate over chemical carcinogens in the USA in order to see what lessons can be learned for Britain. Second, the fact that different regulatory decisions have sometimes been made in Britain and the USA over the *same* chemicals (aldrin/dieldrin or benzene, for example) leads us to enquire into the political context in which such decisions have been taken in Britain. Third, it must also be said that it is often easier for British observers to obtain information about a particular substance from the USA than from British sources. Since regulatory discussions in Britain usually take place under a veil of secrecy, it is useful to investigate the relevant American debates, in order to 'guess' how similar discussions may have been conducted in this country. Finally, it is clear that the present debate over the 'politics of cancer' in the USA will have a substantial impact on future British policies on regulation of carcinogens. Although it now appears that the legislative activities of the European Economic Community (EEC) will become increasingly influential, there can be no doubt that American developments will continue to have important international repercussions.

The regulatory process in Britain and the United States: a comparison

There are striking differences between the British and American systems for the regulation of carcinogenic substances. In the USA, far greater progress has been made in identifying such chemicals and stricter standards have been set for their control. An increasing number of carefully designed animal experiments are now being undertaken, and those chemicals which are shown to be carcinogenic in valid animal tests are officially presumed to pose a cancer risk for humans. Indeed, government agencies, such as the Environmental Protection Agency (EPA) and the Occupational Safety and Health Administration (OSHA), now carry out their regulatory activites on this basis. In Britain, however, the screening and regulation of carcinogens has received very little public, political or even scientific attention. Less animal testing is carried out and the need to control chemicals on the basis of animal data alone has still not been conceded.

The reasons behind these different policies are complex, but one important factor is obviously the scale of the problem. In absolute terms, the American chemical industry is considerably bigger than its British counterpart, particularly in the area of petrochemical production. In 1979, for example, the American industry produced nearly thirteen times more polyethylene and polystyrene, and six times more polypropylene and polyvinyl chloride (PVC) than the British industry, even though the population of the USA is only four-and-a-half times that of Britain.[1] Similarly, an estimated 700 new chemicals are introduced into commerce each year in the USA, compared with between 200 and 400 in Britain.[2] On the other hand, the difference in the number of workers employed is not so great – in 1979, the American chemical industry employed some 1,100,000 compared with 440,000 in Britain. Thus, we cannot explain the greater degree of progress made in controlling carcinogenic chemicals in the USA simply in terms of the larger size of their problem. There are, in addition, a number of social and political differences between the USA and Britain which have been, and still are, especially significant in their effects on carcinogenic regulation policies.

Public participation in the regulatory process

During the post-war period, there has been a growing awareness in the USA of the dangers of many chemicals – both new substances and also those already in use – and this has led to demands for greater public involvement in the relevant decision-making bodies. American environmental and consumer lobbies are larger and more broadly based than they are in Britain. In association with the trade unions, they have been able to use their power to achieve some degree of success in pressing specific arguments related to cancer prevention. In particular, they have monitored the relationship between government regulatory officials and representatives of industry, so as to bring out into the open any collaboration that might develop between the two groups.

By contrast, there are very few organisations in Britain which can claim to represent the broader 'public interest' – certainly none on the scale of the movement in the USA.[3] So far, only the trade unions have managed to exert any degree of pressure on the regulatory process, and even they have varied very considerably in the resources they have chosen to allocate to campaigns over health and safety issues.

The growth of 'public interest' groups in the USA is closely linked to the more open style of regulation and decision-making which has traditionally existed there. An important aspect of this is the Freedom of Information Act which has allowed individuals and groups outside government and industry considerable access to relevant technical reports as well as to statements of intended policy. In addition, federal agencies are required to hold public meetings so as to allow open debate on regulatory questions and on other important public issues. Congress also has a network of subcommittees, whose duties include overseeing the activities of various governmental bodies and scrutinising the general direction of their policies. These subcommittees have the power to call government officials as witnesses before hearings which are usually open to the public; a written record is kept of all transactions. Taken together, these aspects of the American system allow interested parties at least to be aware of the policy alternatives under discussion and to make an independent assessment of the case being made both by the 'regulators' and the 'regulated'. Without such basic information no effective participation by 'outside' groups can take place. Thus, although existing American procedures could certainly be improved, they do at least provide for the possibility of citizen participation and offer the opportunity to influence policy-making at various stages. It must, however, be noted that the American regulatory system is now under attack as a consequence of the changed political climate in that country since Ronald Reagan became president. It is now clear that Reagan's rhetoric of 'deregulation' – freeing business from 'unnecessary restraints' – has substantially weakened the operation of carcinogen controls.

The 'style' of British regulatory activity differs very considerably from that in the USA. Since 1974, the control of workplace hazards has been supervised by the 'tripartite' structure of the Health and Safety Commission (HSC), which includes representatives from industry, local government and trade unions. However, this structure is by no means typical of the rest of the regulatory system, which consists mainly of advisory committees working behind closed doors and in close co-operation with civil servants. Confidentiality appears to be a dominant concern. Consequently, the minutes and proceedings of these committees are never published, the criteria by which they operate are rarely made public, and few detailed reports of their findings and decisions are made available. The committees consist predominantly of supposedly independent experts and virtually no provision is made for 'public interest' groups to be involved in the decision-making process. In addition, committee members are not usually required to disclose any conflicting interest they may have in general or on a particular issue. Unlike the adversarial situation in the USA, the British regulatory system is geared towards the achievement of a consensus between regulators and the regulated. In this way controversy can be avoided and existing assumptions about carcinogenic risks, and how they should be calculated, can survive without 'outside' challenge.

The use of the legal system

In the USA, citizen participation is also facilitated by the structure of the legal system. Claims for workers' compensation and product liability are relatively frequent and high levels of damages from a few cases of the latter have been awarded in recent years. In part, this easier access to the courts stems from the fact that lawyers are generally paid by results on a contingency basis (that is to say, they take a proportion of any damages awarded, up to 33 per cent, but do not charge an unsuccessful claimant), and this provides a major incentive for lawyers to involve themselves. Thus, the judicial system provides one way in which the effectiveness of regulation can be monitored and – where necessary – effectively challenged. In addition, pressure groups have been able to use the courts to petition regulatory activity by the various agencies. Indeed, legal action by 'public interest' groups has been behind many of the regulatory decisions made in the USA in recent years. The Oil, Chemical and Atomic Workers' Union (OCAW), for example, with the assistance of various health pressure groups, helped to push OSHA into issuing its first carcinogen list (of 14 chemicals) in 1974. On the other hand, the legal system can of course be used by industry to obstruct regulatory action. An illustration of this is provided by industry's successful petition in the American courts against OSHA's proposal to lower benzene standards (see chapter 4).

In Britain, the legal system is far less accessible to groups or individuals wishing to influence policy-making. No direct equivalent to product liability exists, and the use of common law is typically cumbersome, slow and extremely expensive. In addition, there is no provision for a 'group' or 'class' action, so that financial responsibility for legal proceedings, has to be assumed by an individual victim. Finally, the rights of groups and individuals in Britain to use the courts to force action by regulatory bodies are virtually non-existent. Generally, then, the British courts have not proved useful as a way of influencing political action over the control of hazardous chemicals.

The collection and dissemination of safety data

The USA is now the major country in the world for toxicological and epidemiological research on the hazards of industrial products and processes. Both state and industrial expenditure on research have increased to cope with recent and anticipated schemes for the regulation of new chemicals. Thus, the American chemical industry has been forced to conduct increasingly stringent toxicological testing before putting new products on the market. Similarly, the federal government has allocated more resources to this area of research. In 1972, total federal government expenditure on environmental health research was in the region of $215 million of which $24 million (some 11 per cent) was spent on research into chemical carcinogens.[4] By 1976, these figures had grown to $485 million and $76 million (15.8 per cent) respectively.[5] When these figures are added to the $500 million spent by industry in the same year,[6] it becomes clear that toxicology, and to a lesser extent epidemiology, have become big business in the USA.

In Britain, the volume of similar research is minute by comparison. In 1977, total government expenditure on toxicological research and training amounted to only about £2 million.[7] Moreover, British toxicology is even more massively dominated by industry than its American counterpart. Industry spending on toxicology amounted to some £50 million in 1977[8] and the vast majority of toxicologists are both trained by industry and work in industry. Many academic toxicologists either receive research funds from industry or are employed as industry consultants. Not surprisingly, therefore, they tend to exhibit a uniformity of approach towards the problem of cancer causation, and this approach often reflects industrial interests. Thus, most British toxicologists take an extremely 'conservative' approach to the identification of carcinogens. They tend to pay little attention to data on animal carcinogenicity and emphasise instead the need to wait for evidence of cancer in *human* subjects before 'proof' can be established – a policy which has been aptly described by several trade unions as 'counting the bodies'.

A serious problem is posed by this lack of British toxicologists who are truly independent of direct or indirect economic links with industry, and who, in other circumstances, could be used by trade unions and other public interest groups to intervene in the regulatory process. In the USA by contrast, a group of toxicologists and epidemiologists who are free of any dependence on industry have been able to challenge industry data and have also been willing to become involved in debates over public policy. The ensuing technical and regulatory controversies have served both to make areas of disagreement overt and also to encourage public education, participation and debate. Indeed, the fostering of this 'critical stance' on questions of carcinogenicity control played a major part in ensuring the ultimate acceptance of the 'generic' approach to carcinogen control adopted by the EPA and other regulatory agencies. (For details, see S. Epstein, *The Politics of Cancer*, Anchor Press (1979).)

In the rest of this chapter we examine the strengths and weaknesses of the British approach to regulating carcinogens in the workplace, in consumer products and in the general environment. If our account appears complicated at times, this reflects both the complexity of the regulatory process itself and also the very low level of public knowledge about what is an extremely important, but almost invisible, area of government activity.

The regulation of carcinogens in the workplace

The history of regulation before 1974

The history of factory legislation extends back to the early nineteenth century when the Factory Acts were introduced to deal with the crisis conditions engendered by the Industrial Revolution.[9] Since then, legislation has been characterised by its partial and fragmentary nature. The 1953 Mule Spinning Regulations, for example, finally prohibited the use of carcinogenic mineral oils only when the industry itself had virtually ceased to exist and some 78 years after the first recorded death of a mule spinner from scrotal cancer. Moreover, no other industries using carcinogenic mineral oils were regulated, even though scrotal cancer was notifiable from the early 1920s and prescribed as a compensatable industrial disease. This illustrates the fact that the British control system has typically been more concerned with compensating the worker than with controlling the original hazards. However, this emphasis should not be taken to mean that Britain actually has an adequate compensation system. The medical panels which assess whether victims of industrial disease are eligible for benefit from the Department of Health and Social Security have come under repeated criticism for their ultra-cautious approach. The pneumoconiosis medical panels are known to reject about 50 per cent of all applications, and the Society for the Prevention of Asbestosis and Industrial Diseases (SPAID) has criticised these panels for their excessively secretive mode of operation.

Cancers induced by nickel, arsenic, wood and leather dusts and benzene are also prescribed industrial diseases (under the National Insurance Industrial Injuries Act) yet the industrial processes using these various carcinogens are not themselves extensively regulated. Thus, by offering compensation, the state recognises the risk to workers. However, it also accepts the continuation of the risk at its existing level and as a result it is the British worker who bears the burden of proof. Such flagrant discrepancies are not due to lack of information, but reflect the influence of industry on the regulatory process and a lack of commitment by government bodies to the removal of unnecessary cancer hazards from the workplace.

The regulations introduced between 1900 and 1974 to control certain categories of a few carcinogens were very limited in their scope. Only four classes of carcinogen were covered over these years – asbestos, aromatic amines, polycyclic hydrocarbons and chromates – and the final two were controlled only in certain sectors of industry. Thus, the Carcinogenic Substances Regulations of 1967 – despite the comprehensiveness implied in the title – dealt only with certain aromatic amines known to cause bladder cancer and used in the dyestuffs, rubber and other industries. The regulations prohibit the manufacture and use in factories of beta-naphthylamine, benzidine, 4-aminodiphenyl, 4-nitrodiphenyl and their salts, *except* when any of these is present in some other material, as a by-product of a chemical reaction in a total concentration not exceeding 1 per cent. Nevertheless, the industrial use of benzidine-based dyes imported from France and Poland has been the subject of a recent trade union campaign in Britain. It is estimated that, despite the regulations, some ten thousand workers continue to handle such dyes each year, and pressure for a total ban on their use has come from the National Union of Dyers, Bleachers and Textile Workers, the TUC General Council, ASTMS, and the Cancer Prevention Society.[10]

The Health and Safety at Work Act 1974
This act deals with all industrial hazards – not just carcinogens – and provides a framework for gradually reforming all previous legislation relating to health and safety at work. For the first time all workers

were covered by a single law and certain provisions were also made for people living near a workplace who might be affected by emissions from it. The Act imposes the general requirement on employers to provide a safe and healthy working environment – but only 'so far as is reasonably practicable'. It also obliges manufacturers, importers, suppliers and designers to ensure that their products are safe by carrying out the necessary testing. They must also supply 'adequate information' relating to the use of the product and to any particular safety precautions which must be adopted. In practice, however, the important phrase 'so far as is reasonably practicable' qualifies all these duties and permits a broad range of compromises between the safety of workers and the expense of safer procedures and processes.

A most important section of the Act allows trade unionists to select shop-floor safety representatives. These representatives can then act for the workforce on health and safety issues and they have the right to request information from their employers on existing and future hazards. Whilst the strength of safety representatives obviously varies between workplaces, the system does at least provide the opportunity for greater trade union influence over the enforcement of safety standards.

The major administrative change enacted by the Health and Safety at Work Act was to bring the various existing inspectorates (i.e. factory, mines and quarries, alkali and clean air, nuclear installations, explosives, agricultural and the Employment Medical Advisory Service) together into one agency – the Health and Safety Executive (HSE). Policy was then delegated to another new body – the Health and Safety Commission (HSC). The HSC is built on a tripartite principle with equal representation from the trade union movement, employers, and local authorities, but its secretariat is drawn from the HSE – i.e. from civil servants. This tripartism also applies to the advisory committees which operate within the HSC for the establishment of safety standards and codes of practice, the most important being the Advisory Committee on Toxic Substances (ACTS; see appendix 8 for membership of this committee). The advisory committees prepare recommendations for the HSC itself (usually after an advisory committee working party has been formed), and these recommendations are often published as consultative documents and criticism and comment invited. The HSC then carries out further consultation with interested parties before returning the matter to the relevant advisory committee. However, at each stage in the regulatory procedure, every attempt is made by HSC and HSE officials to achieve some kind of consensus and to iron out major disagreements *before* a consultative document appears. Thus, in sharp contrast to the explicitly adversarial and open nature of the American system, this ensures that at least an appearance of unanimity continues to be maintained. However, its weakness is that an intransigent party can block attempts to reach any decision at all, thereby seriously delaying the whole regulatory process.

The control of carcinogens and other toxic hazards since 1974
The British HSC/E have as yet no official policy for the regulation of carcinogens. Indeed, the HSE insists that control of carcinogens should be subsumed under the general control of toxic chemicals. The HSE used to point to one of its publications, *Toxic Substances: A Precautionary Policy* (1977) as its major statement of intent. This four-page document argues the case for an overall plan for the control of the potential carcinogens only in the most general terms:

> When a substance is known to cause cancer in humans, rigorous control measures, including prohibition where appropriate, are essential and their implementation is enforced at all times. When a substance is suspected of being carcinogenic, increasingly strict control measures are taken concomitant with the available evidence of carcinogenicity.[11]

However, the document gave no detailed guidance as to precisely what such control measures might involve. So far, the HSE has itself set only four carcinogen control standards – for vinyl chloride (VC), acrylonitrile, benzene and asbestos.

It has recently become clear that there is some difference of opinion within the occupational health and safety authorities (or rather between the HSC and the HSE) over the creation of a *specific* policy for occupational carcinogens. The Advisory Committee on Toxic Substances set up the Carcinogens Working Party, in 1978, which drafted proposals for separate regulations for the control of carcinogens – but these proposals have never been published. In 1982, however, the HSE published a so-called technical report (*Carcinogens in the Workplace*),[12] written by H. J. Dunster, Deputy Director General of the HSE, in which he expressed the view that the HSE 'hopes to move towards a *single comprehensive* set of regulations dealing in fairly general terms with the control of substances hazardous to health' (emphasis added). Carcinogens would simply be

> subject to the more stringent requirements of the regulations . . . the more certain it appears that a substance is or will be a human carcinogen and the more potent a carcinogen it appears to be, the more stringent will be the control requirements, but the process of identification as a carcinogen will not take the substance out of one control regime into another.

This report, and the philosophy underlying it were strongly criticised by several trade unions since it appeared to be a firm statement that carcinogens would not be treated differently from other toxic substances; yet no such policy had been agreed by the tripartite HSC which is supposedly responsible for broad policy matters of this kind. The HSC promptly dissociated itself from the report, claiming (in March 1982) that 'policy for control of all substances hazardous to health (including carcinogens) for use at work is under consideration by the Commission who expect to issue a consultation document in due course'.[13]

It would seem, then, that there is some degree of confusion and disagreement within the state regulatory authority over how potential carcinogens should be controlled. But however these disputes are resolved, it is also clear that there is a further obstacle to setting new and more adequate safety standards. This stems from the lack of accurate information about the carcinogenic effects of many industrial materials on either animals *or* humans. As Edward Langley of the Hazardous Substances Division of the HSE pointed out in 1978, 'the testing of industrial and commercial chemicals in the past has been rudimentary and directed primarily toward the acute effect rather than the chronic.'[14] Similarly, industry has usually carried out systematic testing only when there is a legal requirement – in the case of food additives or drugs, for instance – but not for industrial chemicals. In recent years, however, experiences with VC in particular have led to serious concern about the safety of many of the chemical industry's most widely used products. They have also demonstrated the crucial importance of testing materials on animals rather than insisting on the delaying and often impracticable tactic of investigating these problems exclusively on humans. This has posed two separate but interconnected problems for the HSE. First, what should be done about carcinogenic or untested materials already in use, and, second, how should the safety of new chemicals be assessed?

The assessment of chemicals already in use
So far there has been no systematic attempt to review the hazards of the 20,000–30,000 chemicals already in commercial or industrial use in Britain. HSE policy is that industry has the legal duty to test these materials under section 6 of the Health and Safety at Work Act, and that firms will notify them of any toxic hazards that are discovered. However, it is open to some doubt whether firms will do this without explicit legislation. It was recently revealed, for instance, that Coalite Chemical Products Ltd had misrepresented the results of a survey into the effects of the highly toxic and carcinogenic dioxin (TCDD) on the workers in their 2,4,5-T plant.[15] In addition, sections of the report (commissioned by the firm in the aftermath of the Seveso explosion) were not made available to either the HSE or the trade unions concerned.

Neither the HSE nor the various state-supported research institutions in Britain are involved in systematic animal research to explore the carcinogenic and other effects of materials in widespread use. This is in contrast to the activities of the National Cancer Institute (NCI) and National Toxicology Program (NTP) in the USA, which have been carrying out a 'bioassay program' of animal cancer tests on major industrial chemicals. This independent testing has had a significant effect in re-evaluating the hazards of certain materials that had previously been considered 'safe' on the basis of either chemical industry testing or even mere assumption. The American NIOSH (National Institute for Occupational Safety and Health), although a separate research agency, in part acts as the research wing of the enforcing agency OSHA. In 1980, it spent about one-fifth of its $50 million budget on research into carcinogens. It has produced over eighty criteria documents reviewing the scientific evidence on hazards of particular chemicals and industrial processes, and recommending precautions and control standards as a basis for regulation. In addition to epidemiological surveys, NIOSH has also carried out a national occupational hazard survey, for 1972–74, which covers 5,000 plants employing over a million workers; it is embarking on a second survey of this type. The British HSE, by contrast, has no developed research wing equivalent to NIOSH. Work is contracted out to the Medical Research Council, but on a much smaller scale, and the only current systematic research programme is attempting to validate short-term cancer screening tests. The HSE does not have – and does not seem to want – the resources to perform the kind of research work in which NCI, NTP and NIOSH have been engaged.

The regulation of new substances
Like most industrialised countries, Britain has at last begun to draw up schemes for pre-market testing of industrial chemicals. In the USA, comprehensive legislation of this sort has already been enacted (the 1976 Toxic Substances Control Act (TOSCA)), although it has not yet been adequately implemented. In the EEC such 'notification' procedures have been adopted in the form of the 'sixth amendment' to the 1967 EEC directive on the classification, packaging and labelling of dangerous substances, and this scheme has now been adopted for implementation in Britain. The HSC, in 1981, proposed a stronger scheme than that derived from the sixth amendment but, after strong industry opposition, was obliged to abandon it.

In brief, the sixth amendment requires that companies wishing to market new chemicals within the EEC must supply the following information at least 45 days before sales commence:

- a technical dossier containing evaluations of the hazardous potential of the chemical concerned;
- a declaration of its 'unfavourable effects';
- proposals for classification and labelling;
- recommended precautions for safe use.[16]

The technical dossier must give various chemical details – such as formula and purity – as well as estimates of quantities to be produced, proposed uses and storing and handling procedures. It must also include the results of some short-term animal tests – acute toxicity (LD_{50}), skin and eye irritation and a sub-acute 28-day exposure study. Also required are the results of two short-term tests for the substance's carcinogenic potential (one using bacteria and one using some other such system).

The details of the scheme were the subject of much negotiation, and British officials had considerable success in getting their 'flexible' approach to pre-market testing adopted. This was in marked opposition to the Dutch who wanted a stricter scheme similar to the American TOSCA.[17] Obviously, any scheme for notification is an improvement on the present situation and therefore welcome, but the EEC scheme has serious inadequacies. These can be seen most clearly if it is compared with TOSCA.

(1) TOSCA's requirements on testing are much stricter than those of the EEC scheme. All notifiable chemicals (that is, those to be produced in quantities greater than 1 tonne per year) have to be subjected to full animal testing, including long-term tests for carcinogenic effects. Under the EEC scheme, requirements for such long-term testing are, in effect, at the discretion of the regulatory authority (in Britain, the HSE). Such discretion is only likely to be exercised if the chemical is to be produced in very large quantities (over 1,000 tonnes per year).

(2) TOSCA requires the publication of information on chemicals provided by the manufacturer to the enforcing agency – in this case, the EPA – so that the information can then be subject to public scrutiny. However, under the EEC scheme, publication of the technical dossiers is at the discretion of the regulatory agency. This discretion was strongly supported by the HSE on the gounds of preserving 'commercial secrecy', though as ASTMS rightly pointed out:

> The chemical companies have no secrets from one another; each can analyse the products of its rivals within hours in an analytical laboratory. The real object of 'commercial secrecy' is to keep information out of the hands of the unions.[18]

(3) Manufacturers have to notify the EPA 90 days in advance of marketing the chemical, giving the EPA plenty of time to require further tests. The EEC scheme allows 45 days (and indeed the HSE argued for only 30 days).

(4) TOSCA gives the EPA the power to ban a hazardous chemical outright. There are no such powers under the EEC scheme, though they may be included in a future set of EEC regulations on the control of toxic substances.

TOSCA was only enacted in the USA after a bitter six-year struggle against the opposition of American manufacturers who eventually succeeded in modifying the thrust of some of its requirements. However, the EEC scheme is even more acceptable to European chemical companies than a TOSCA-style one would be. Indeed the HSE, reflecting the views of the British chemical industry, are of the opinion that too vigorous pre-market testing requirements would actually impede innovation. Their 1977 discussion document on the subject of notification alleges (without supporting evidence) that the £12,000–20,000 (in 1977 prices) cost of carrying out the minimum toxicity texts (i.e. *excluding* tests for carcinogenicity and mutagenicity) 'would cause the abandonment of many projects – perhaps 30–50 per cent of the total'.[19] It might well be asked whether products which do not justify the spending of such relatively small sums of money on basic testing are worth developing at all.

Early in 1981, the HSC, in response to the requirements of the sixth amendment to the EEC directive, published a revised and more extensive scheme (*Notification of New Substances*, consultative document),[20] which included the basics of the EEC scheme with two principal additions. First, chemicals produced during a production process which are not themselves the final product, but to which workers might be exposed (so-called 'intermediates') would also be included in the notification regulations. Toxic intermediates would therefore have to be notified to the HSE and full assessments of their toxicity might have to be produced. Second, included for notification in addition to obvious industrial chemicals would be pharmaceuticals, food additives, pesticides and tobacco substitutes. Although these substances were already regulated by other committees, the HSE might require further information on them for the purpose of assessing their toxicity to *workers* rather than just to consumers.

Industry, particularly the pharmaceutical industry and those firms represented by the CIA, was vehemently opposed to these additions, arguing that they would lead to higher costs and would put the British chemical industry at a disadvantage compared to its European rivals. The refusal of industry representatives to agree to the HSC's proposed scheme led the HSC to abandon it in late 1981 (though a 'working party' was set up to examine particularly contentious issues). The weaker EEC scheme was therefore adopted instead.

It is important to stress one major consequence of the comparative laxity of British (and European) testing requirements. American firms will be attracted overseas – where pre-marketing requirements are much less stringent – for the initial marketing of new chemicals. Thus, if control procedures in this country are not brought up to American standards, there is a danger of Britain becoming a testing ground for 'dirty' chemicals.

The overall conclusion must therefore be that, inasmuch as they necessitate some pre-market testing for new chemicals, the EEC notification schemes do represent an advance on the existing situation. However, they can only be a tiny step in the political struggle to reduce public exposure to carcinogens.

The regulation of carcinogens in consumer products

The Department of Trade is responsible for the safety of all consumer products used in and around the home which are not the specific concern of other government departments. The main products falling outside their jurisdiction are pharmaceuticals, which are regulated by the Department of Health and Social Security (DHSS), and food products and pesticides, which are both under the supervision of the Ministry of Agriculture, Fisheries and Food (MAFF). Under the Consumer Safety Act of 1978, the Secretary of State has, for the first time, the power to prohibit the supply of any dangerous goods which appear on the market, and also to insist that hazardous consumer products which are already available should be the subject of published warnings. Within the department itself, the Minister of State for Consumer Affairs takes special responsibility for consumer protection and information and also for product liability. So far, two prohibition orders which relate to carcinogenic substances have been made under the 1978 Act. These concern children's nightwear treated with the flame retardant chemical Tris and balloon-making compounds containing benzene.[21]

The most striking features of the British system for the control of known or suspected carcinogens in consumer products are the diversity of the regulatory authorities concerned and the lack of public participation in the process. These can be illustrated most effectively by reference to three types of product – food additives, medicines and pesticides.

Food additives
Under the Food and Drugs Act of 1955, it is illegal to sell food which is either 'unsound' or 'injurious to health'. A special section of the Act (part V) covers regulations dealing with food additives and contaminants. These regulations list permitted additives according to their function (e.g. preservatives, artificial sweeteners and colouring agents), and specify the permitted levels for each substance. The devising and amending of the permitted lists are the responsibility of MAFF, which acts on the recommendations of the Food Additives and Contaminants Committee (FACC). FACC is a committee of experts and does not include formal representation from interested parties – either the food industry or the general public. However, it should be noted that many of the experts serving on FACC are, or were until recently, employed by companies concerned with food manufacturing, such as Smedley–HP, ICI, Unilever and Reckitt and Colman. (For membership of this committee see appendix 9.)

When an additive is considered by FACC, recommendations are made on the basis of two explicit criteria – need and safety. The judgement of 'need' may be based on a range of factors including either supposed 'consumer demand' or the potential of the relevant chemical for solving technical problems faced by the food industry. The onus is on the manufacturers themselves to submit evidence of both need and safety. In principle, strictly economic criteria are excluded from the discussion of need, but, in practice, it appears inevitable that the economic interests of companies are paramount in their decision to introduce a new additive. Moreover, because FACC basically functions 'behind closed doors', a full and open discussion of various assessments of 'need' is impossible. In such circumstances, there is a distinct danger of a close and friendly relationship developing between the regulators and the regulated industries. This means that industrial claims about the potential social utility of a product can continue without external challenge.

Medicinal products

The thalidomide tragedy of the early 1960s suddenly brought to public attention the lack of any systematic procedure in Britain for the testing and clearance of drugs. The 1968 Medicines Act was designed to remedy this situation by establishing a system within the Department of Health and Social Security (DHSS) for the granting of clinical trial certificates, product licences and permission to market new medicines. The day-to-day operation of the Medicines Act is carried out by the medicines division of the DHSS and by a series of advisory committees. The most important of these are the Committee on the Safety of Medicines (CSM), which gives advice on applications for licences of new drugs, and the Committee on the Review of Medicines (CRM), which considers those products which are already on the market. Both committees are composed of independent experts and do not include any wider public representation.

Broadly speaking, British controls over the safety of medicines are more systematic and stringent than those for any other type of consumer product. The DHSS has produced a series of '*Notes for Guidance on Carcinogenicity Testing on Medicinal Products*', which specify those occasions when such testing should be conducted and lay out broad principles for the form that toxicological studies should take. However, the Association of the British Pharmaceutical Industry (ABPI) has been involved in lengthy negotiation with the DHSS and its relevant expert committee over these guidelines. While the original notes for discussion (published by the DHSS in September 1977) stated that carcinogenicity testing should be carried out where a substance would be administered to humans for any period greater than six months, the ABPI argued that this period should be extended to twelve months. After protracted negotiations this longer period was eventually accepted by the DHSS. There has also been an important debate between the pharmaceutical industry and the DHSS over the number of species to be included in carcinogenicity testing. The ABPI claims that one species alone is sufficient, while the DHSS have argued that two species must be involved.

These negotiations over carcinogenicity testing illustrate the fact that although such decisions may *appear* to be purely technical, they are in fact taken within a wider political and economic context which cannot be ignored. Clearly, the pharmaceutical companies have a strong interest in maintaining their profits, and therefore will be likely to oppose any regulatory policy which they see as expensive to themselves. We have already seen, for instance, that they opposed pharmaceuticals being included under the HSC's proposed scheme for pre-market assessment of chemicals to which *workers* are exposed. However, as in the case of food additives, the relevant advisory committees and decision-making bodies are structured in such a way that the results of testing are not made public and economic and political arguments of this kind cannot be explicitly debated. Rather, they operate on the basis of an assumed – but mythical – consensus between government regulators, the regulated industry and consumers, a situation which can lead to a disregard for the wider public interest.

Pesticides

The efficacy and safety of pesticides is under the control of MAFF. Efficacy is assessed by the Agricultural Chemicals Approval Scheme and a list of approved products is published each year. However, there is no legal restriction on the sale of unapproved products. Safety is regulated under the Pesticides Safety Precautions Scheme (PSPS) which was created in 1957. It functions through the Advisory Committee on Pesticides (ACP), consisting of ten academics and civil servants, with a scientific subcommittee of technically qualified civil servants and academics, who review all pesticide applications. (For membership of ACP see appendix 10.)

Four grades of clearance are available for pesticides, from limited trials to full commercial clearance – all based on chemical, toxicological and usage data supplied by companies. An impressive list of toxicological requirements is given in an appendix to the PSPS handbook, but in practice companies only carry out tests as they see fit.

PSPS is voluntary, inasmuch as no individual firm is forced to join it. However, once the decision to join has been made, the firm is then obliged to be bound by government decisions. The scheme has been reinforced by the British Agrochemicals Supply Industry Scheme (BASIS), under which agricultural merchants undertake to sell only those products cleared by PSPS. In turn, members of the British Agrochemicals Association (which initiates the manufacture of about 95 per cent of the active ingredients of all pesticides marketed in Britain) have agreed to supply only those companies that are members of BASIS. In practice, however, the voluntary nature of the scheme, and the lack of worker or consumer representation on the appropriate committees has led to widespread criticism of the pesticide regulatory scheme (see especially chapter 6).

The regulation of carcinogens in the general environment

Mechanisms for regulating environmental pollution and carcinogens in Great Britain are similar in character to those we have already examined in relation to consumer goods. That is to say, they are complex and fragmented and provide little or no opportunity for independent experts or concerned citizens to participate in the regulatory process. Indeed, both these criticisms probably apply even more in the area of environmental carcinogens than elsewhere.

To begin with, there are at least six separate pieces of legislation which form the basis for this area of regulatory activity.

(1) Alkali, etc., Works Regulation Act, 1906 This consolidated existing legislation on environmental pollution. However, it specifies actual emission limits for only three processes;[22] for all others, the idea of 'best practicable means' is used as a basis for regulation, although operating guidelines and 'presumptive standards' do exist.

(2) Health and Safety at Work Act, 1974 This imposes a general duty on manufacturers to use the best practicable means to prevent

fugitive emissions from a workplace into the environment of local communities.

(3) Public Health Acts, 1936 and 1961; Public Health (Recurring Nuisances) Act, 1969; Public Health (Scotland) Act, 1897 These lay out the responsibility of local authorities for pollution control.

(4) Clean Air Acts, 1956 and 1968 These acts extend the provisions of the Public Health Acts in regard to smoke nuisances. However they relate only to those processes which are outside the jurisdiction of the Alkali Inspectorate.

(5) Control of Pollution Act, 1974 This allows local authorities to obtain full information about emissions from industrial premises.

(6) Road Traffic Acts, 1972 and 1978 These acts regulate the constitution of fuels used in motor vehicles and are supervised by the Department of Transport.

The above breakdown of legislative provisions illustrates the extremely confusing and fragmented nature of the British framework for pollution control. Moreover, these laws govern a wide range of different kinds of environmental contaminants (e.g. air, freshwater, marine, noise and solid wastes), and the responsibility for implementing them is divided between a large number of government departments and regulatory bodies. Government agencies involved in the control of environmental pollution include the following:[23]

1 Cabinet Office – interdepartmental decisions
2 Department of Transport – vehicle emissions
3 Department of the Environment – general co-ordinating functions and responsibility for policy in a number of areas
4 Ministry of Agriculture, Fisheries and Food (MAFF) – protection of fisheries and responsibility for Pesticides Safety Precautions Scheme (PSPS)
5 Department of Trade (DoT) – marine pollution
6 Department of Industry (DoI) – industrial and economic aspects of pollution
7 Department of Health and Social Security (DHSS) – provides medical advice, especially through its Committee on Carcinogenicity of Chemicals in Food, Consumer Products and the Environment

8 Department of Energy – advises on nuclear installations
9 Department of Employment – responsibility for health, safety and welfare of persons at work
10 Health and Safety Commission (HSC) – responsibilities under the Health and Safety at Work Act, 1974
11 Department of Education and Science (DES) – funds basic science through its research councils
12 Foreign and Commonwealth Office – international implications of environmental policies
13 Ministry of Defence – supports various types of relevant research
14 Scottish Office and Welsh Office – various environmental responsibilities in their respective countries
15 Royal Commission on Environment Pollution (RCEP) – advises on national and international matters concerning the pollution of the environment

This division of responsibilities is further complicated by the lack of clarity concerning the functions undertaken by each agency. Thus, in the case of research for example, the Department of Industry has three relevant research establishments (Warren Springs Laboratory, the Laboratory of the Government Chemist and the National Physical Laboratory), whilst the Department of Education and Science also funds environmental analysis through its research councils (particularly the National Environment Research Council). Other agencies may also sponsor research related to a specific environmental problem. So far as policy-making is concerned, initiatives may come from almost any of the above agencies – although the Royal Commission on Environmental Pollution and the Department of the Environment play an especially significant role. Similarly, advice for future policy may come from any of the listed agencies. Overall, then, it is very difficult if not impossible to characterise the specific function of each institution – each operates on a flexible basis and each is able to play a role in research and policy-making according to the particular circumstances.

The complexity of the system is further exacerbated by the fact that *regulatory* duties are not concentrated in any one body and even the responsibility for one specific type of pollution can often be divided between various departments – as we show below with reference to air pollution. The fragmented and even chaotic nature of the British regulatory system is best illustrated by comparing it with the American situation, where the EPA combines most of the responsibilities listed above in a single authority. Such a model is undoubtedly more efficient, allowing for the creation of a general policy rather than a piecemeal and incremental approach to the problem of controlling environmental carcinogens.

An additional feature of the British system is that it frequently grants an individual department the conflicting responsibilities both for regulating an industry and also for promoting its growth. The Department of Trade, for example, in addition to stimulating British export sales and promoting general economic growth is also responsible for controlling oil pollution at sea. This creates an obvious danger that the development of a close working relationship between government officials and industry representatives will discourage the establishment of stricter environmental standards. Thus, MAFF has been criticised for being concerned more with the profitability of farms than with the health and safety of agricultural workers. In the USA, 'public interest' groups have paid particular attention to situations of this kind, where there is conflict of interest and the possibility of an agency being 'captured' by industrial interests. In Britain, however, such problems have received little or no attention.

The Alkali Inspectorate: a case study

As an example of the British control system in practice, we now look at the regulation of air pollution by the Alkali and Clean Air Inspectorate (AI).

The AI was originally created under the 1906 Alkali, etc. Works Regulation Acts. Since its transfer from the Department of the Environment in 1974, the AI has been located within the HSE. It has responsibility for air-borne emissions from some two thousand 'registered works',[24] other emissions being largely the responsibility of local authority Environmental Health Departments (EHDs). The division of responsibility between the AI and the EHDs is made partly according to mere tradition and partly on the principle that the AI should deal with the more complex and problematic types of emission control. Fundamental to the AI is its 'special relationship' with the industries which it regulates. As a recent Royal Commission Report commented:

> The essence of their approach lies not in standing back from the industry but, on the contrary, in being intimately involved in it. The Inspectorate collaborate closely with the industry in seeking solutions to pollution problems.[25]

Central to this approach is the use of the important concept 'best practicable means'. That is to say, national air quality standards have been rejected in favour of a case-by-case strategy as outlined by a former chief alkali inspector:

> There must be a compromise between: (1) the natural desire of the public to enjoy clean air; (2) the legitimate desire of the manufacturers to meet competition by producing their goods cheaply and therefore to avoid unremunerative expenses; and (3) the overriding national interest.[26]

The operation of 'best practicable means' has been succinctly described as being rather like 'a good system of contract bridge played with a co-operative partner'.[27] This regulatory approach is geared towards the achievement of a compromise between factory owners and the local inspectorate. Although general guidelines are provided by 'presumptive limits', the system is highly flexible and the emission controls imposed on any individual workplace are the result of a process of negotiation. The economic effects of regulation on a factory are therefore taken into account by the alkali inspectors although explicit cost-benefit analyses are rarely carried out.

Quite obviously, the alkali inspectors are given large discretionary powers under this system. Unfortunately, however, these powers are not balanced by any degree of accountability to local communities. Although there are provisions under the 1974 Control of Pollution Act for local authorities to obtain accurate information on pollution, and to make this available in a public register, such information has rarely been provided. Moreover, the AI has not tended to be helpful to individuals in search of details about specific emissions. Indeed one chief alkali inspector has recently referred to media coverage of pollution issues in the following terms: 'Mischievous and exaggerated publicity . . . can cause fears in the public and introduce gulfs. It can also lead to social problems, unrest and militancy.'[28]

In the light of comments of this kind, it is perhaps not surprising that the AI's attitude to the public was itself criticised as follows in a recent Royal Commission Report:

> To the public whose interests they serve they sometimes appear remote and autocratic. There has been some clumsiness and insensitivity in the Inspectorate's public pronouncements and an air of irritation with those who presume to question the rightness of their decision.[29]

Thus, in contrast to the situation in the USA, public knowledge about environmental pollution is sparse, and it is very difficult to discover even what standards are being used to regulate carcinogens. Following the recent EEC directive, regulations are now being developed which will provide the public with information on the hazards of new substances about which the manufacturers will be required to notify relevant authorities such as the Department of Environment. However, notification of this kind is likely to be of little value if it merely states that the 'authorities' consider a substance to have certain hazards without giving details of the reasons for that conclusion or specific proposals for control. Meanwhile, the secrecy of the British system has encouraged various 'public interest' groups to demand a greater degree of public participation in the control of environmental pollutants (for details of some of these groups, see appendix 7). Whilst the 'contract bridge' approach may be acceptable to the two partners concerned, it is inevitably unsatisfactory for those outside who may well suffer the consequences of any decisions that are made and therefore not unreasonably wish to be included in the decision-making process itself.

Conclusion

We have seen that in contrast to the USA, the procedures for the regulation of carcinogenic substances in Britain are generally fragmented and conducted in private. They operate on the basis of consensus between government-appointed experts rather than the more adversarial, open and participative approach which has developed in the USA. The only exception to this is the regulation of workplace hazards where, after a long history of piecemeal reform, the Health and Safety Commission and its advisory committees now operate on a tripartite basis. This system has given one 'public interest' group at least – trade unions – a right both to be heard and, equally importantly, to hear and challenge the views of government officials, industry representatives and medical and scientific experts. However, this system is far from perfect in practice. Although the HSC has held 'public hearings' (when it was collecting views regarding the control of asbestos in the late 1970s), most of its decision-making processes are not open to public scrutiny.

Finally, it is important to emphasise that there is a clear distinction between the process by which standards for exposure to toxic and carcinogenic substances are set and the mechanisms by which these standards are then implemented and enforced. Despite its various deficiencies, the American standard-setting system is superior to the British equivalent. However, in the area of the enforcement of those few standards which exist, the British system appears more effective – at least so far as the workplace is concerned. Thus, the number of inspectors per workplace and their legal powers are greater in Britain, particularly since the 1974 Health and Safety at Work Act. The USA therefore has more satisfactory standards, but less effective means of enforcing them, whilst the UK has less adequate standards, but more effective enforcement – though the British Factory Inspectorate is currently experiencing financial cut-backs.

This situation illustrates the serious defects of the policies being practised in *both* countries and the critical need for sweeping reform. It is particularly important that the *relatively* greater effectiveness of the enforcement procedures in Britain should not be used as a justification either for not improving the regulatory system itself – which has serious faults – or for leaving standards at their present unsatisfactory level.

4. Case studies: the workplace

Introduction to the case studies

In chapters 4, 5 and 6, we provide case studies of twelve individual carcinogens found in the workplace, in consumer goods and in the general environment. Our initial choice of chemicals was dictated by the contents of Epstein's *Politics of Cancer* and our aim was to compare the regulatory history of the various substances in Britain and the USA. We have also added an additional example – 2,4,5-T – because of its particular relevance to the current debate about regulation in Britain. However, constraints of time and space inevitably mean that our coverage is still very partial. For instance, we do not cover the tragedy of bladder cancer in workers exposed to aromatic amines in the dyestuffs manufacturing and rubber industries. This is the subject of another book. Nor do we cover the history of cancer in the town gas manufacturing industry, where hundreds of workers have died of lung, bladder and kidney cancer caused by the retort house fumes. Other cases of occupational cancer have also been omitted – lung cancer from nickel manufacturing fumes, for instance, scrotal cancer from pitch and tar and the many types of cancer caused by radiation.

Our intention is that the case studies should illuminate the workings of the British regulatory system, demonstrating, in particular, the social and economic influences on what are often represented as purely scientific decisions. We also see the case studies providing clues about how the regulatory process could be strengthened – a theme that we pursue in more detail in our concluding chapter.

Asbestos

Despite conclusive evidence of the grave hazards of asbestos, the production, processing and sale of asbestos-based products remains big business. Annual world production exceeded 6 million tonnes in 1978, compared with only 2.25 million tonnes in 1960. The British share of asbestos processing is, however, declining. From a peak of nearly 200,000 tonnes imported into Britain in 1973, imports in 1979 were down to 117,000 tonnes.[1] But the British asbestos industry is still worth some £200 million and employs over 20,000 people, while at least another 100,000 came into regular contact with asbestos in their daily work.[2] Asbestos continues to be incorporated into a very large number of products, many in everyday use at home and at work.

Three companies now dominate the UK asbestos industry – Turner and Newall, Cape Industries, and British Belting Asbestos – and their profits could be said to have been achieved at grave human cost. Between 1969 and 1976, 1,189 people employed in asbestos-related industries in the UK were diagnosed by pneumoconiosis boards as suffering from lung fibrosis or asbestosis, and were therefore eligible for compensation. Similarly, between 1957 and 1975, some 1,952 people were officially admitted to have died from mesothelioma, a cancer of the chest or abdominal lining, and the vast majority of these must have contracted the disease through occupational exposure to asbestos.[3] Asbestos has also been clearly implicated in other cancers, particularly of the lung and gastro-intestinal tract. It is important to remember, however, that those figures represent only the tip of an iceberg since there is certainly a massive under-reporting of the death and disease caused by asbestos.[4] Between 1968 and 1977, for example, 388 death certificates recorded both asbestosis and lung cancer. Lung cancer is not prescribed for compensation and this would only be awarded if the pneumoconiosis medical panels accepted that the degree of asbestosis present had materially accelerated death. If the same degree of asbestosis is accompanied by another cancer (e.g. cancer of the pancreas), the death is not recorded as asbestos-related at all. The cancer, not the asbestosis, is held responsible for the death and no compensation is paid. The exception to this is the cancer, mesothelioma, which *is* prescribed for compensation. However, although it is accepted that nearly all mesotheliomas are due to exposure to asbestos, very few are *officially* recognised as arising from occupational exposure. For example, out of 328 cases of mesothelioma in 1977, only 88 (that is 27 per cent) were awarded industrial death benefit.[5] Thus the total number of deaths from exposure to asbestos is not officially investigated or recorded, but epidemiological surveys show that lung cancer is now the most significant cause of deaths induced by asbestos. If this is taken into account, it is likely that there are now about 2,000 asbestos-induced deaths each year.[6]

The hazards of asbestos and the failure of existing regulations to deal with asbestosis were highlighted by TV documentaries in 1975–76 and a report was published by the parliamentary commissioner (or ombudsman) in 1976.[7] The ombudsman had been asked by a former worker suffering from asbestosis to investigate the situation at the Acre Mill asbestos plant in the Yorkshire village of Hebden Bridge. In his ensuing report, the ombudsman emphasised the dangers of working with asbestos and criticised the Factory Inspectorate for their failure to enforce regulations regarding effective safety measures. Some 2,200 workers had been employed in the mill from its opening in 1939 to its eventual closure in 1970. More than 260 of these workers (12 per cent of the total) have already developed asbestos-related diseases, and, according to a local doctor, at least 59 *of those workers he could trace* had died of such diseases by 1978, 44 of them from lung cancer or mesothelioma.[8]

The situation at Hebden Bridge must be considered against the general background of the history of asbestos regulation in Britain. Though a Home Office report had pointed out the dangers of asbestos as early as 1906, it was not until 1928 that government research into the problem was undertaken. It was then found that as many as four out of every five workers who had spent more than 20 years in the industry were suffering from asbestosis. Cancers were not looked for. These revelations resulted in the introduction of a set of regulations in 1932 to control levels of asbestos dust in a limited number of asbestos factories.

However, the regulations were pursued with little vigour and proved markedly ineffective. Indeed, only *two* prosecutions were ever undertaken during the period of almost 40 years that the regulations were in force. The 1950s and 1960s saw a marked increase in the number of asbestosis cases in asbestos textile factories as well as in other asbestos-processing industries and amongst those workers using asbestos, who were not then covered by the regulations. The relation between asbestos and lung cancer, first recorded in 1938,[9] was confirmed by Doll in 1955. Mesothelioma, a rare cancer of the stomach or lung lining, was confirmed in asbestos workers between 1960 and 1964 and subsequently found in people decades after they had been exposed to relatively low concentrations of asbestos dust for only short periods. Cases among relatives and neighbours illustrated how far this carcinogen had penetrated into the wider community.

The official response to these discoveries was the introduction of new asbestos regulations in 1969. These regulations extended controls over asbestos dust levels to include those working with asbestos products, while a technical data note recommended that exposure to asbestos dust should not exceed two fibres of white asbestos (chrysotile) per cubic centimetre of air. This particular level of exposure was justified on the grounds that it would 'reduce to 1 per cent the risk of getting asbestosis through having worked for a life time with asbestos'.[10] The process by which this standard came to be set illustrates with particular clarity the way in which economic criteria have been – and still are – major determinants of regulatory decisions of this kind.

The 1969 standard was set following the advice of a committee of nine members of the British Occupational Hygiene Society (BOHS), four of whom were from the industry-financed Asbestosis Research Council. The data upon which the standard was based came from a study by company doctors and scientists at Turner and Newall's Rochdale plant. This study was based on an examination of workers in only one factory, and only workers employed for at least ten years *and still there* were included in the study. Of the 290 that were examined for signs of asbestosis, eight (3 per cent of the total) were initially found to have the disease. However, there were serious deficiencies in this study. First, no follow-up was undertaken of those workers who had left the works or even those who had died – a proportion of whom were likely to have had asbestosis. Second, asbestosis can take up to 20 years or longer to develop, so that many of the workers surveyed would not yet show signs of the disease. Conversely, many of those who had been there *less* than ten years would have received enough exposure to develop the disease later but were excluded from the survey. Finally, the study considered only asbestosis, and excluded mesothelioma and other cancers known to be related to asbestos exposure. It was thus entirely predictable that the survey would underestimate the incidence of asbestos-induced diseases. That it did so was confirmed by later follow-up studies when asbestosis was found in 140 workers, or almost 50 per cent of the original sample.[11] By 1972, Turner and Newall confirmed that ten of the original 290 had died of lung cancer or mesothelioma, a rate far higher than expected in the general population.[12] Thus, the evidence on which the 1969 standard was based is of very dubious scientific value. But even if the data had been adequate, it is still unclear why the committee should have considered a 1 per cent risk acceptable. Why not a 0.1 per cent risk, or 0.01 per cent or no risk at all? Obviously, economic criteria were most important here, a view which is supported by the comment of one asbestos-industry member of the subcommittee that: 'It is important to take into account the economic consequences of any recommendations made as well as the benefits for health.'[13]

Even when the inadequacies of the original data were subsequently revealed, the subcommittee still made no recommendations for change. For largely commercial reasons, the asbestos companies had settled on two fibres per cubic centimetre as a standard they wanted. It was convenient that the scientific data appeared initially to support such a standard, but when subsequently they did not, no changes in the standard followed. (The Report of the Advisory Committee on Asbestos (ACA) in 1979 later confirmed that the medical data used for the 1969 standard had underestimated the incidence of the disease by about fifteen times.)[14]

Despite all these efforts, public demands for greater control over exposure to asbestos were rekindled by events at Hebden Bridge. As a result of this concern, the HSC set up the tripartite Advisory Committee on Asbestos, in 1976. The 1977 interim statement of the committee simply reaffirmed the existing unsafe exposure limit. However, in its final report, presented in October 1979, the ACA took the unusual step of proposing three different 'control' limits for the three principal forms of asbestos (for membership of this committee see appendix 11). Under this scheme, the standard for blue asbestos (crocidolite) would remain at the 1969 level of 200,000 fibres per cubic metre (0.2 fibres per cubic centimetre, which is roughly approximate to daily inhalation of as many as 1.6 million fibres), the standard for brown asbestos (amosite) would come down from 2 million fibres per cubic metre (2 fibres per cubic centimetre) to 500,000 fibres per m^3 (0.5 fibres per cubic centimetre) and the standard for white asbestos (chrysotile) would come down from 2 million fibres per m^3 (2 fibres per cubic centimetre) to 1 million per m^3 (1 fibre per cubic centimetre). In proposing these new limits, the ACA rejected demands for a phased ban on asbestos put forward by the TUC. In his evidence to the advisory committee, an independent epidemiologist, Julian Peto, projected that even a 1 fibre per cubic centimetre limit for white asbestos would lead to 2 per cent excess mortality from lung cancer and 2 per cent from mesothelioma – in addition to the 1 per cent excess from non-malignant respiratory disease.[15] This totals 5 per cent excess mortality overall, or one extra death in every group of 20 workers, a risk that is apparently judged as 'acceptable' by the ACA.

Only one of the 53 recommendations of the ACA report had been implemented by the beginning of 1982. Even the proposed licensing laws for the asbestos-removal industry, which had been the subject of a special ACA interim report in 1978 calling for 'urgent action', had been blocked by the Confederation of British Industry (CBI) and the HSE, who did not want to legislate in advance of EEC directives proposed in 1980. Then, in July 1982, Yorkshire TV screened 'Alice – A Fight For Life' – a dramatic documentary which concentrated on the cancer hazards and in particular the mesothelioma hazard still associated with asbestos. Public reaction forced the government to implement key ACA recommendations on control limits, on licensing the asbestos removal industry, and on the prohibition of certain products and processes. Following pressure from the unions, the HSE announced further reviews of the medical evidence, and of control methods, with a view to lowering the control limits still further in 1983–84. These issues are also being investigated by the Commons Select Committee on Employment, following parliamentary pressure organised by the GMWU and SPAID (for details of SPAID, see appendix 7). The risks to non-asbestos workers and to the general public from asbestos products in the workplace and the community have so far received very little attention. However, the unions and the Institute of Environmental Health Officers have now demanded an end to the misapplication of the asbestos *occupational control limit* to non-asbestos workers and the public, and the use instead of an *environmental control limit*. In the absence of an official environmental control, the GMWU has proposed a limit of 5,000 fibres per cubic metre (0.005 per cubic centimetre) for any type of asbestos.

Asbestos has already caused the deaths of thousands of people, and may cause another 50,000–70,000 deaths in the next 30 years.[16] Removing the millions of tons of asbestos in the community will either cost the taxpayer in excess of £1,000 millions, or will cause even more deaths if the job is done dangerously. Laws on the prevention of asbestos-related diseases and the compensation of victims have been on the statute book for 50 years, yet the tragedy continues. The detailed history of this failure of control has yet to be written, but it is clear that a new approach to dealing with occupational carcinogens is necessary if this history is not to repeat itself. However, the attitude now being adopted by employers and the HSE towards the 'man-made' mineral fibres (MMFs), particularly fibre glass, increasingly being used to replace asbestos does not augur well for the future. Enterline in the USA and Sarracci in Europe have both identified excess respiratory tract cancers in manufacturing workers exposed to very low concentrations of some of those substances over 30 years. This reinforces positive animal data that have been available for over a decade, yet an HSE working party's recommendation to halve the MMF-control limit, published in 1980, had still to be implemented by December 1982.[17]

Benzene

Benzene is one of the most widely used organic chemicals and about 1.14 million tonnes are produced in Britain each year. It is an important raw material within the chemical industry, as well as being a commonly used solvent found in petrol, paints and printing inks, as well as in a wide range of other consumer products. It has long been recognised that exposure to benzene can cause blood abnormalities, particularly aplastic anaemia and leukaemia (a cancer of the white blood cells) but benzene poisoning did not become a notifiable industrial disease in Britain until 1966.

In the 1950s, the British Threshold Limit Value (TLV) was set at 25 parts per million (ppm), but in 1969 it was reduced to 10 ppm, following the lead of the American Council of Government and Industrial Hygienists (ACGIH). (For explanations of TLV and ppm measurements, see appendix 12.) In 1972, the Factory Inspector's Medical Division (the forerunner of the Employment Medical Advisory Service) published guidance notes on the use of benzene, specifically mentioning its leukaemogenic (leukaemia-inducing) properties and damaging effects on chromosomes. By 1975, it was recommended that the use of benzene in school laboratories should be discontinued. A year later, the HSE recommended that the industrial use of benzene should be discouraged, and that workplace controls should reduce atmospheric concentrations as far below the 10 ppm standard as possible.

In April 1977, OSHA, after accumulating further evidence of benzene's leukaemogenic properties, proposed its emergency standard of 1 ppm, but the HSE failed to follow suit and an HSE official commented, 'to the best of our knowledge there has been no evidence of any new threat to health.'[18] The HSE's Advisory Committee on Toxic Substances (ACTS) then reviewed the evidence on benzene's toxicity again in 1979, on the basis of an EMAS review paper, and decided not to lower the 10 ppm standard. Typically, the review was confidential and anonymous. It also failed even to analyse the substantial recent data that exist both on benzene's carcinogenic properties and also on its chromosome-damaging effects at concentrations below 10 ppm. This review was subsequently rejected by the TUC representatives on ACTS while

ASTMS had the following comments to make on the review's quality:

> The word 'leukaemia' was used *once* in this review, and that in a reference to a paper by Jandl (no source given) stating that in 1977 'no cases of leukaemia arising in workers exposed to benzene had been reported in American literature since 1961'. Well! either the EMAS has completely misunderstood this reference, or Jandl is sadly mistaken . . . *One* other study of chronic effects of benzene is cited, by Pagnotto (again no source) to the effect that some workers exposed to benzene in the rubber coating industry showed no signs of blood disorders. *Out of the literature running to scores of papers and several reviews, the vast majority of which report positive findings of a link between benzene exposure and leukaemia, the HSE 'review' paper selects two reports, unsourced, which give negative results.* And on the basis of this, the Advisory Committee find that there is 'no evidence' to support lowering the current control limit.[19]

The trade union side on ACTS have since demanded that the benzene standard be reconsidered and that a TLV of 1 ppm should be enacted (to bring the control into line with the standard demanded by OSHA).[20] They argue that the evidence linking leukaemia with benzene is incontrovertible.

Stung by these rebukes, EMAS looked again at the health effects of benzene, and produced a more substantial paper running to nearly eighty pages.[21] This paper accepted the toxicity of benzene in the blood system, and its mutagenicity, carcinogenicity and teratogenicity at relatively high doses (around and above 100 ppm). However, the review went to great lengths to avoid accepting direct evidence that benzene induces these effects at lower dose levels – and in particular at levels below the current TLV of 10 ppm.[22] EMAS apparently believed that a threshold level can be demonstrated for carcinogens – a view that flies in the face of independent scientific opinion as expressed by a wide range of official bodies, including the World Health Organization's (WHO) International Agency for Research on Cancer and the International Commission on Radiological Protection, as well as NCI, NIOSH and OSHA.

The efforts of EMAS to deny that there is direct evidence of the carcinogenic effects of benzene at levels around 10 ppm are misleading. Even discounting the evidence of such effects below 10 ppm, the fact that it is known to cause effects at 100 ppm is sufficient, *for regulatory purposes*, to infer that it causes one-tenth or some other fraction of the effects at 10 ppm. For these reasons, trade union representatives have continued to press for more stringent control over benzene.

Events in the USA in 1980, however, made the trade union position more difficult. The 1 ppm benzene standard promulgated by OSHA in 1977 was rejected by the Supreme Court in July 1980.[23] This standard had been debated at public hearings held through the summer and was finally ratified in February 1978, but it was challenged in the courts by industrial groups, who claimed that OSHA had failed to demonstrate that there would be 'significant' public health benefits flowing from the new regulation. After a New Orleans district court granted a stay to these industrial interests, the case went to the Supreme Court where the decision was upheld by a five-to-four majority. It spelt out its reasoning in an important series of statements. First, it should be noted that neither the lower court nor the Supreme Court queried the fact that benzene causes leukaemia or that thresholds cannot be set for carcinogens. Nor did the Supreme Court uphold the decision of the lower court that OSHA need consider the cost–benefit ratio of any new measure. This would delay regulation by several years and the Supreme Court wisely threw it out. What the majority of the Supreme Court did find, however, was that OSHA had failed to establish that benzene 'poses a significant health risk in the workplace, and that a new lower standard is therefore reasonably necessary or appropriate.' The four minority judges entered a very strong dissenting judgement, saying that the decision flagrantly disregarded restrictions on judicial authority, and took the court into areas of dispute that it could not expect to resolve (i.e. scientific and medical controversies). The minority concluded that the decision was nothing less than an attempt to deny the federal authorities the right to act to curb a *presumptive risk*. In other words, they would have to wait until there were dead bodies on show before a substance could be said to pose a 'significant' hazard.

There can be no doubt that this Supreme Court decision weakened the bargaining position of both American and British workers in their efforts to reduce the allowable limit for benzene exposure. However, the campaign was given new urgency by the recent publication of a study of benzene workers conducted by NIOSH.[24] Out of 748 workers exposed to benzene in two American factories making rubber hydrochloride in the 1940s, at least 7, and possibly up to 11, had died of leukaemia by 1975 (only 1 or 2 would normally have been expected to contract the disease). Although some of these workers had been exposed to benzene concentrations of several hundred ppm, for the most part the benzene levels to which they had been exposed fell within the limits permissible at the time of the exposure (that is, below 100 ppm). Indeed, in one case the benzene level was as low as 16 ppm – not far above the current TLV of 10 ppm. The study argues in conclusion that 'benzene is a human carcinogen at a range of exposures not greatly above the current legal standard' – a view that implies that the current TLV is too high, and that the campaign to reduce it needs to be continued.

Vinyl chloride (VC)

Vinyl chloride (VC) has achieved a certain notoriety as the first of the chemicals of the modern plastics age to be clearly and publicly linked with cancer. The chemical first became industrially important in the 1930s when its ability to polymerise was exploited in the manufacture of the plastic polyvinyl chloride (PVC). After the Second World War, production of PVC steadily increased to the extent that it is now one of the most common and widely used plastics in the world. In Europe alone, annual production is around 5 million tonnes per year of which something in excess of 400,000 tonnes is produced in Britain, almost all of it by ICI.[25]

The PVC is made by heating VC gas in solution with small amounts of other chemicals under pressure. After a certain period the polymerisation reaction becomes uneconomically slow and the pressure vessel is cleaned out and reloaded with a fresh mix. The PVC slurry, still containing some unreacted VC, is dried and the PVC (usually in granular form) sent off to a fabrication plant to be made into one of its many end products.

Hazards known from an early stage to be associated with this production process are the flammability of VC gas and its ability to knock workers out at high concentrations. Throughout the 1950s and 1960s evidence of other problems grew. The most obvious symptom of exposure was a bone deformity called acro-osteolysis, which caused clubbing of the fingers; other symptoms included violent mood change, intense itching and painful numbness of the limbs. There was also some evidence of liver damage resulting from chronic exposure.[26] In the light of the evidence on acro-osteolysis, a TLV of 200 ppm was set in Britain. Many of the workers in PVC production plants did receive high doses of VC, particularly those who had to climb inside the pressure vessels to chip solidified PVC off the walls between loads.

In 1970, the first report of cancer in animals exposed to VC gas was made by P. Viola, a toxicologist, who had exposed experimental rats to 30,000 ppm VC.[27] Following Viola's results, a group of European producers commissioned a more detailed study by the Italian toxicologist Cesare Maltoni. By late 1972, his preliminary results showed cancers in various organs in rats, mice and hamsters and, as his trials continued, he discovered that these cancers were still caused even at levels of exposure as low as 50 ppm. One particularly rare form of liver cancer – angiosarcoma of the liver – was especially noticeable.[28] European companies then started to study their own records to see if there was evidence of excess cancers among their workers. Subsequent research in the USA led to a startling announcement by B. F. Goodrich: in 1974, this company revealed that three workers from their PVC plant in Kentucky had died of liver angiosarcoma since 1971. Following this announcement, the American exposure standard was reduced from a TLV of 500 ppm to 1 ppm and, despite threats that this would be too expensive, the industry fairly quickly managed to tighten control of the production process so as to achieve it, and in so doing made substantial economies.

In Britain the events which followed the announcement were very important for the history of the regulation of occupational hazards, since they provided an early test of the principles of the 1974 Health and Safety at Work Act. When the Act was first introduced it had considerable support from industry. The consensus approach which was enshrined in the Act meant that industry itself, in consultation with government and unions, would have a powerful role in determining safety standards and procedures. Thus, when the tripartite committee of industry, government and union representatives (the VC Working Party) was formed to discuss a new VC standard, there was considerable pressure from the chemical industry to agree quickly to an 'economically practicable' level. Indeed, the speed with which this apparently democratic approach produced the new standard of a 10 ppm eight-hour average was cited by the Chemical Industries Association as a vindication of the consensus method itself:

> Thanks to the commonsense approach of the UK authorities and the concerted efforts of the companies, effective control procedures have been achieved in the UK without the UK companies being subjected to the counter-productive difficulties which have plagued the industry in the USA.[29]

In fact, this 'commonsense' approach meant that the standard arrived at was largely based on the levels of VC which industry claimed they could hope to achieve in the workplace air. Criticism of the apparent laxity of the standard compared, say, to the proposed new American standard of 1 ppm was answered by pointing out that the standard arose from a tripartite agreement, and that, in any case, it would be more strictly implemented than the standard set in other countries, including the USA.

However, there was a small but outspoken opposition which argued that the standard was too lax for such a potent carcinogen. Furthermore, dissenters argued that the apparent agreement between industry and labour representatives in the tripartite discussion was largely a reflection of the control exercised by the companies over relevant information and the consequent paucity of data available to trade unionists. Members of the British Society for Social Responsibility in Science (BSSRS), for instance, were involved in a community project on pollution around British Petroleum's Baglan Bay plant. They were surprised by the BP workers' complacency on VC and their ignorance of the extent of its possible hazards. Although BSSRS initially encountered some suspicion from the workers, and were strongly opposed by the management throughout, they were ultimately able to convince the workers of the risk and helped them to bargain with the company to force the concentration of VC in the air down below the 10 ppm standard.[30]

A great deal of publicity was generated by a BSSRS TV programme and by science journalists concerned about the secretive and apparently lax approach adopted in Britain towards carcinogens; industry was forced to marshal a substantial public relations campaign. This again was something of a departure from previous practice, but industry was not entirely unprepared. This was mainly due to ICI, who belatedly recognised the possible significance of the problem. Although a quick check of their own mortality records had revealed no cases of angiosarcoma, ICI were already alarmed by at least seven cases of primary liver cancer (some subsequently diagnosed as angiosarcoma) identified in Europe and the USA before the Goodrich cases were made public. They persuaded the CIA to set up a committee to cope with the problem.[31]

This CIA committee was mainly responsible for proposing a code of practice on PVC manufacture, for representing the industry in its tripartite discussions, and for coping with any public relations problems. This latter activity consisted largely of trying to play down the problem by concentrating on the rarity of angiosarcoma of the liver, denying the induction of a wide range of other cancers by VC as unproven, and stressing the low exposure levels of all but a few people who worked in polymerisation plants. The committee was critical of groups like BSSRS who were said to prevent the possibility of a 'reasonable' approach and were described as 'the grit which slows down the machine'.[32]

It is important to realise that the HSE code of practice is concerned solely with the manufacture of PVC and, even at its inception, applied to only six plants: ICI Hillhouse Works, near Blackpool; ICI Castner Kellner Works, Runcorn; Vinatex Stavely Works, Chesterfield; BP Chemicals, Baglan Bay, South Wales; BP Chemicals, Barry, South Wales; and British Industrial Plastics, Aycliffe, near Durham. Recently the number has become even smaller as BP is pulling out of PVC production so that its Baglan Bay works and all but one plant at Barry, which is being taken over by ICI, will be closed. (The closures have nothing to do with the hazards of VC, but are part of the general shake-up in the European chemical industry to reduce its current over-capacity.) The far more widespread processes of fabricating finished PVC products from raw PVC are not covered at all, despite the fact that VC can be released from PVC under heat or pressure. Moreover, the tripartite approach to regulation does not extend to the problem of VC release into the general environment. In this country the most significant sources of such exposure are loss of unreacted VC from finished PVC products, and emissions from VC and PVC plants. These are the responsibilities of the MAFF and the AI, respectively.

Many foodstuffs are packaged in PVC. Bottles for cooking oil and fruit drinks, margarine tubs and flexible wrapping for meat and vegetables can all be made of PVC. In 1978, MAFF's Steering Group on Food Surveillance published a report which stated that VC concentration in packaging and hence in food was greatly reduced over the period 1974-77.[33] Their estimate was that maximum daily intake per person was reduced from 1.3g in 1974 to 0.1g in 1977. They concluded by praising the success of co-operation between government and industry and made no recommendations for further change. In other countries, however, concern has been shown even at the very low levels which currently exist. In Italy for instance, use of PVC bags as containers for blood and its separated factors was suspended in 1978.

The AI's approach to vinyl chloride pollution in the air has been very similar. The HSE report on industrial air pollution for 1976[34] (published in 1978) reveals that the AI had adopted a provisional target for emissions of 2.4 kg for every tonne of PVC made in the six plants covered by the code of practice, and that two plants were exceeding this target. The report does not name them but merely says that the two problem plants are those in which a dispersion grade PVC (of finer particle size than ordinary suspension grade) is made. The only numerical details given in the report concern a relatively new practice for the AI of monitoring the air around the plants rather than emissions from the plant. The figures for the Vinatex plant are given as 63 per cent of readings less than the limit of detection (0.005 ppm), 97 per cent less than 0.034 ppm and the highest daily value (out of 215 samples) was 0.12 ppm.[35] For comparison, in the USA the Environmental Protection Agency calculated that the average exposure of the 4.6 million people who live within five miles of PVC manufacturing plants was 0.017 ppm in 1974–75, and it has been concerned to reduce such figures by 95 per cent.[36]

In 1978, the EEC issued a council directive[37] on VC to harmonise regulation throughout its member states. The directive covers not just VC and PVC manufacturing workers but also any workers 'exposed to the effects of vinyl chloride monomer in a working area'. The directive also differs from the present standard in this country in that the standard employed is a 'Technical Long Term Limit Value' (TLTLV) which says that exposure to VC should not exceed 3 ppm when averaged over a whole year. In addition to the year-long average, however, there are various 'action levels' for shorter periods of time, the idea being that if an action level is being exceeded then steps should be taken to reduce exposure right away. For instance, the action level for an eight-hour period is reckoned to be 7 ppm.

Clearly, the British regulations do not meet the requirements of the directive, and will have to be changed. At the time of writing (June 1982), the VC working party of the HSC had not been reconvened to discuss the changes required and it seems likely that the HSE will overcome this problem simply by adopting the more complicated TLTLV standard of the EEC directive wholesale, and using it as the 'control level' for VC in the new list of standards being prepared to replace the TLV list. This reluctance to reconvene the tripartite VC working party may well be due to the fact that the new proposals would not have such an easy passage, as the trade union representatives are now better informed and more determined to get the lowest possible standard.

In addition to the much stronger line they are taking on standards, trade unions have also been demanding better medical monitoring, and, at ICI, workers have demanded a compensation scheme which recognises cancers and other diseases in workers exposed to the high pre-1974 levels. In 1980 a group of workers from Vinatex's Stavely plant received compensation totalling £750,000 for 'VC disease', the general term for the non-carcinogenic symptoms of exposure to VC.[38] To prevent claims for civil damages from reaching the courts, ICI and BP have now produced their own compensation schemes and the ICI scheme covers both angiosarcoma and fibrotic liver damage.[39]

The significance of the VC issue thus far has been threefold. First, in Britain, as in the USA, it demonstrated that, despite what they usually claim, in this case companies could stand the cost of regulation without appreciable losses. (The cost of engineering improvements in the UK up to 1978 was estimated at £15 million.) Thus the often quoted threat that more regulation would mean fewer jobs was not a real one. Second, and very important, information coming from outside the formal regulatory process was taken up and used by trade unionists in an attempt to reduce their health risks by collective bargaining. Third, it demonstrated once again the predictive power of animal data and helped to establish the case for basing regulatory action on non-human evidence – a corner-stone of the new approach to occupational carcinogens now being recommended by unions and concerned scientists. Fortunately, the human evidence on VCM was 'discovered' shortly after the animal evidence and the tumour concerned was rare – had it been lung cancer, the VC story would have been much more protracted. As it is, however, IARC now recognises that VC also causes lung cancer and cancers of the haematopoietic system, but the unions have so far failed to convince employers or the HSE of this.[40]

Acrylonitrile (AN)

Acrylonitrile (AN) is manufactured in Britain by Monsanto at Seal Sands, Teesside and by BP Chemicals at Grangemouth on the Firth of Forth. Its main use is in the manufacture of acrylic fibre, but it is also quite widely used with other chemicals in the manufacture of a range of plastic moulding materials, such as acrylonitrile-butadiene-styrene (ABS), which are used to make containers for foodstuffs and cosmetics.

In January 1977, the American Manufacturing Chemists' Association reported preliminary results of an animal study they had commissioned which showed carcinogenic effects from AN in drinking water at levels of 100 and 300 ppm. Results later that year revealed that the effects also occurred at far lower levels (35 ppm in drinking water, 20 ppm by inhalation). Further, in May 1977, Du Pont Chemicals made public the results of an epidemiological study of a group of 470 workers at an acrylic fibre plant in south Carolina which revealed a higher than normal incidence of lung and colon cancer.[41] Within a year, the American regulatory agencies had taken steps to reduce the workplace exposure standard and to reduce the risk of consumer exposure – for instance, by the banning of AN-based plastic bottles for Coca Cola.[42]

In Britain, however, events moved more slowly. Immediately after the news of the Du Pont study reached Britain, ASTMS held a meeting with the CIA. At this meeting, in June 1977, the CIA argued that there was no need for a specific standard for workplace exposure – though without producing any figures for current exposure levels in British industry. The TUC then referred the matter to the HSC's Advisory Committee on Toxic Substances who first discussed it in August 1977. Progress at this and subsequent meetings was slow. Initially, there was much debate over just what the levels of exposure to AN were in British plants. The CIA argued that it was difficult to take accurate measurements below 2 ppm and that there were also problems with the use of different measuring techniques by different companies. Even when more accurate figures were eventually produced, in 1978, discussion of a new standard was further delayed because the companies had not produced estimates of the cost of controls.

But the response of the chemical industry was not solely one of passive resistance. The CIA had already set up a working party – the Acrylonitrile Health Impact Study Team (ANHIST), consisting of industrial hygienists and manufacturing experts – in February 1977, three months before the problem was first picked up by ASTMS. ANHIST operated on several fronts. While on the one hand arguing for a voluntary standard for exposure to AN of 10 ppm (half the existing TLV that had been set on the basis of short-term hazards only), they also attempted to play down the hazard. Working jointly with the HSE, they initiated an epidemiological study of 1,111 workers exposed to AN in British plants. It revealed a slight excess of deaths among the workers. In particular a cluster of 5 stomach cancers were found among workers from Welsh factories and an excess of lung cancer in 15–44-year-olds was also noted.

However, they decided that the overall cancer increase was not statistically significant; that the Welsh stomach cancer may have been due to some regional rather than occupational factor, and that in the absence of information on smoking habits, the lung cancer could not be definitely linked to AN. A spokesman for Monsanto (UK), Alec Munn, who was at the time the president of the British Occupational Hygiene Society, stated on TV, in June 1978, that 'It has not been demonstrated that for man, at least, any level [of AN exposure] is particularly dangerous other than in terms of acute poisoning.'[43]

Such a statement was very misleading. At that time, the positive results from both the Du Pont study and the animal experiments had been available for more than a year. Not surprisingly, therefore, the position adopted by Monsanto (UK) and other British firms came under attack from the unions – notably ASTMS. Indeed, criticism even came from the American chemical company Du Pont, whose spokesperson, Charlie Mullikin, expressed scepticism about the British AN companies' opposition to implementing a 2 ppm standard; Du Pont, he pointed out, had achieved that level in a plant that was considerably older than any in Britain.[44]

When ACTS did reach a compromise recommendation for a 4 ppm standard, it was rejected by the Confederation of British Industry's representative on the HSC. However, in May 1979, the HSC eventually agreed to a 5 ppm standard, which would be reduced to 4 ppm in 1980 and 2 ppm by 1981. Thus, the 2 ppm standard for workplace exposure to AN was introduced into Britain three years after it had been adopted by OSHA and, despite the chemical industry's objections, the level appears to have been achieved without too much difficulty.

The AN story is one example of the way industry can offset the cost and inconvenience of regulation by using delaying tactics. One such tactic was to plead that the cost of achieving the 2 ppm limit would be impossible to meet, and then to take over 12 months to say that they could not produce an estimate because they needed a control limit as a basis on which to work out the costs. Since the control limit itself was the central issue in dispute, this brought the argument round full circle. Arguments about exposure levels, about the relevance of animal data, and about uncertainties of epidemiological findings were also used to spin out the discussions on ACTS.

The arguments over the AN control limit also provide perhaps the clearest illustration of the way in which the 'dirty end' of an industry dictates where the employers' side will seek to establish the control limit – even where the majority of users can achieve a much lower control limit. Exposure records showed that over 90 per cent of the industry could achieve a 2 ppm limit for AN in 1979, but one particularly 'dirty' plant could not, and its position had to be protected by the negotiating stance taken by the CBI. Since that time, the unions have found that, for a number of substances, a small 'dirty' part of an industry has dictated the control limit level. This has applied in the case of asbestos, styrene, formaldehyde, glass-fibre, and carbon disulphide, in particular.

Why was industry so anxious to avoid reductions in the control limit when fewer than 2,000 workers were directly exposed in the making and processing of AN? The answer seems to be concern about the possible public relations problems that would stem from another cancer scare about a substance which was widely used in the packaging of a variety of consumer products. We have already seen that, in the USA, considerable attention had been given to the use of AN plastics in food-packaging and Monsanto had been adversely affected by the ban on plastic Coca Cola bottles.

If that was a concern, then the industry need not have worried. It has taken the various committees involved a long time to deliberate on the issue in this country, but eventually, in April 1982,[45] they decided that *no action* was necessary to restrict the use of AN materials for food-packaging, despite the decisions taken in the USA. As was the case with VC, the Steering Group on Food Surveillance decided that the industry was doing enough to bring down levels of AN in food. For instance, they claimed that the amounts absorbed by people eating soft margarine (in AN plastic tubs) had fallen sharply between 1975 and 1979 as a result of changes in the production process. Therefore, despite the decision from the Committee on Carcinogenicity of Chemicals in Food, Consumer Products and the Environment that the evidence was 'at least compatible' with the conclusion that AN caused human cancer, the government report concluded that co-operation between industry and government had once again proved valuable and that 'the general public are not at measurable risk from AN in food'.

Bischloromethyl ether (BCME)

In 1948, a small chemical plant opened in Pontyclun, near Cardiff. It used chloromethyl ether (CME) to make ion exchange resins for large-scale users of water such as electricity generators and steelmakers. During this process, formaldehyde and hydrochloric acid are combined, yielding bischloromethyl ether (BCME) as an intermediary, and as a 1–7 per cent contaminant of CME. During the First World War, both France and Britain had rejected the use of BCME as a poison gas because it was too volatile and unpredictable. In 1949, in the USA, the Dow Chemical Company enclosed a similar process because of the well-known ability of CME to cause intense lung irritation. Their chief chemist was well aware of the potential hazard in 1948, and his views at that time were quoted by a Dow executive in 1973:

> I'd like to share with you a posture taken some 25 years ago . . . which definitely recognises CME as a severe respiratory irritant and called for handling methods similar to those recommended for radioactive materials. I propose to continue work on the semi-plant production and use of CME to make anion exchange resins on the basis that all equipment be installed by external controls. If such operation proves impractical I believe we should abandon large-scale work with chloromethyl ether.[46]

These precautions by Dow greatly reduced the exposure of their workers to the two chemicals. Unfortunately, similar precautions were not taken at the South Wales plant, nor at the American plant owned by the USA's other major producer, Rohm and Haas. Workers at both plants were to pay a high price for this management 'oversight'.

In 1962, the Rohm and Haas company doctor noted an excessive number of lung cancers in one part of the plant at Bridesburg. After a careful study, management concluded that CME was the most likely cause of the excess lung cancers.[47] They were advised to commission some animal testing of their chemicals to see which was responsible and they approached Dr Norton Nelson, a leading lung cancer expert. Dr Nelson and the company apparently could not agree on the terms under which the research would be conducted.

However, Rohm and Haas finally contracted Hazleton Laboratories, who confirmed, in a preliminary report in 1966 (and in a slide-show presentation to managers in February 1967), that both CME and BCME were carcinogenic in mice. One group of mice exposed to BCME at 10 ppm had died within five days – most survivors had lung tumours. These results were not published at the time. However, it is significant that in that same year Dow Chemical recognised BCME as a human carcinogen and fully informed their employees.[48] Meanwhile, Dr Nelson had secured federal funds for research on BCME and in 1968 his team reported their preliminary findings because, they said, 'of high carcinogenic potency of BCME already apparent in studies still underway'. They advised that, 'extreme caution be exercised with respect to skin and inhalation exposure'.[49] In 1969, Dr Nelson's team confirmed their preliminary results. Another study, this time in mice, showed lung tumours caused by BCME.[50]

By the end of 1969, there was very clear animal evidence on the carcinogenicity of BCME in two species of animals, but some of it had not been published. Moreover, Rohm and Haas had investigated their clinical suspicions of 1962, and had found an eightfold excess of lung cancer in the 35–54 age group at their Bridesburg plant,[51] but again they did not make this public for several years. However, it seems likely that this information was passed on to the Rohm and Haas management at their UK plant near Newcastle since engineering controls at that plant kept exposures to BCME much lower than at the Permutit plant at Pontyclun in Wales. The Permutit plant was the only other UK factory making BCME – yet they seem to have been unaware of the mounting evidence of the cancer-causing properties of BCME.

In October 1969, the observant GMWU shop stewards at the Pontyclun plant, Andrew Tree and Des Roberts, noticed that 'too many' of their workmates had died of lung cancer. Some had died at suspiciously young ages and some were non-smokers. They wrote to the union about their suspicions, enclosing a list of 20 chemicals used at the plant, including CME and BCME. The letter was passed to Dr Murray, who is now a freelance occupational health consultant, but who was then the medical adviser to the TUC. In his reply, he said that 'in the list of chemicals indicated in the letter of 20th October, none is likely to have been the cause of cancer.'[52]

In 1971, further animal evidence confirmed that CME, and particularly BCME, were extremely potent carcinogens, causing 'startling tumour yields (lung and nasal cancers) at extremely low concentrations',[53] which made them 'extremely hazardous in industrial handling'.[54] In the same year, the evidence showing animal tumours from inhalation at exposures as low as 0.1 ppm was presented to the British Occupational Hygiene Society's Fourth International Symposium.[55] However, from discussions with the Pontyclun workers who were at risk from BCME every day, it seemed that they were not yet aware of its dangers. In the USA, the human and animal evidence accumulating was sufficient to bring about a meeting of over a hundred representatives from the ion exchange industry, from academia and from the government to discuss the implications of the evidence. The meeting took place on 22 July 1971. Dr Norton Nelson, whose team had established the startling animal evidence, was in no doubt about the conclusion of their meeting: 'No reasonable person could have left that meeting without the knowledge that we were dealing with a potent carcinogen, a very nasty substance indeed.'[56] The American occupational health authority, NIOSH, began their own epidemiological study of BCME. The news of the meeting in the USA, and the evidence presented to it, must have reached Britain because, in August 1971, an attempt was made to clean up and to reduce exposures to CME and BCME at the Pontyclun plant. An epidemiologist from Newcastle University, Dr McCallum, was asked to do a mortality survey of the workforce. At the same time, the medical department of the Factory Inspectorate began its own epidemiological survey under Dr Owen, who is now the TUC's medical adviser.

In October 1971, Andrew Tree wrote to the GMWU again, noting the American animal evidence and the one case of nasal cancer that had occurred at the Pontyclun plant; nasal cancer had also been identified in the animal studies. Dr Murray replied, saying that the nasal cancer

> might be due to occupational exposure but at the same time it might just be one of those cases which occasionally arise in the general population . . . I think the only thing to do is to continue with the remote control of the process at the present time and await further evidence from Dr McCallum's researches.[57]

He was later to acknowledge that at the time of this second reply 'the toxic and carcinogenic properties [of BCME] were unknown to me.'[58]

However, less than 12 months later, the American Conference of Governmental Industrial Hygienists (ACGIH) concluded that there was sufficient evidence to classify BCME and CME as human carcinogens, and published this in their 1972 list of threshold limit values for toxic substances. The Factory Inspectorate, on publishing this list in the UK (as they had done every year since 1965), formally endorsed this conclusion. In the same year, some human evidence was published for the first time in an American health and safety newsletter.[59] In addition, 'preliminary formal, but unpublished studies were completed (at the USA plant of Rohm and Haas) between 1971–3 . . . lung cancer rates were significantly higher for the entire plant.'[60]

Meanwhile, in Pontyclun, Andrew Tree was still failing to convince 'the experts' that his members were at real risk from BCME. Following his third enquiry, a meeting was arranged in June 1972, at the factory. It was addressed by Dr Murray, Dr Owen, Dr McCallum and local Factory Inspectorate representatives. The men recall that the impression given was that animal evidence was not to be trusted and that the human evidence was not convincing enough. After all, as Dr Murray pointed out in his report on the visit,

> cancer of the lung is so common in the general population as a result of cigarette smoking that it would need very strong evidence to be able to attribute the cases arising in the factory to any other environmental cause.[61]

In May 1973, a year later, the lung cancer rate at the American Rohm and Haas plant was confirmed to be eight times the normal rate, in a published study by a local doctor, Dr Figueroa.[62] He had noticed the excess of a particular type of lung cancer, and, on enquiring into the cases, traced the pattern back to the Rohm and Haas plant. Figueroa compiled a study on the basis of data collected from the workers and from his own medical records. It turned out to be remarkably accurate. Human evidence was now piling up. Three other epidemiological studies were published that year confirming the carcinogenicity of BCME.[63]

However, the first British human evidence was found to be entirely contrary to all the animal and human evidence gathered elsewhere. Dr McCallum had finished his study of the Pontyclun plant in April 1973, and his most significant conclusion was that 'the study does not support the hypothesis that there has been exposure to a carcinogen.'[64] The strangest thing about this study was the epidemiological methods used. In order to identify excess cancer in a workplace, it is usual to compare the cancer rate in the workforce with the cancer rate in the rest of the country. Dr McCallum, however, compared the cancer rate in the *whole of the local area* (Llantrisant and three other wards) with that of the rest of the country. Not surprisingly, he found no excess of cancer. The Pontyclun workforce would have needed to be very large, and/or the cancer epidemic huge for it to have elevated the cancer rate amongst the thousands of people living in the local communities. The technical manager at the time confirms the view held by the men that McCallum's study reassured everyone:

> I have no memory of the details of the survey but it appeared reassuring at that stage, and I copied a sentence from the covering letter which said 'you will see that we do not find any evidence of an increased cancer mortality which one might expect where there is a cancer hazard in the factory.'[65]

The local Factory Inspectorate continued to apply their relatively relaxed policy to the company, not insisting on total enclosure, nor even on the continuous monitoring of the workplace atmosphere, precautions which the American plants had adopted two years earlier.[66] It was to be 1982 before continuous monitoring for BCME leaks and exposures replaced the weekly 20-minute grab samples that had been the sole scientific measure of exposure at the Welsh plant until then. And it was not until 1982, after the union's insistence, that adequate cancer warning signs were displayed in the plant.

Dr Murray and EMAS both knew of Dr McCallum's negative evidence when it was reported to the company in 1973. However, it appears that no effort was made to tell the union, the company, or the men that the study was methodologically flawed, or that the scientific human evidence which they had all been waiting for had in fact been established beyond doubt by 1972 when ACGIH, NIOSH and HSE declared CME and BCME carcinogens. In 1974 OSHA confirmed that CME and BCME were human carcinogens. At about the same time EMAS decided not to continue with its own epidemiological study of the Welsh plant because the human evidence was so overwhelming that further evidence, especially from a small study, was unnecessary.[67]

Unfortunately, EMAS did not tell the company or the men of this fairly significant policy decision. When the American company, Diamond Shamrock, took over the Pontyclun plant in 1977 they were unaware that their workers were the subject of a half-finished epidemiological study. Meanwhile, the Pontyclun workers were still left with 'the experts'' view that their lung cancer problem was more likely to be caused by smoking, and with Dr McCallum's conclusion that they were not exposed to a carcinogen.

By 1976, more human evidence had accumulated,[68] and Dr McCallum, on hearing of the abandonment of their study, asked EMAS if he could finish it for them. His 1973 conclusion clearly needed updating; EMAS agreed, but did not provide any of the funds to do it.

In 1979, Dr Owen, now at the TUC as their medical adviser, sent the protocol (i.e. the description of methods and procedures) for McCallum's proposed completion of the EMAS study to David Gee, National Health and Safety Officer of the GMWU. Gee sent it to the Pontyclun plant, asking if the stewards knew about the proposed study. At a special safety committee meeting in January 1980, Diamond Shamrock, the new owners of the Pontyclun plant, acknowledged the existence of Dr McCallum's 1973 study (no copies had been given to the workers), and sent it to the Chemical Industries' Association for their views. Dr Howard, the CIA medical adviser, considered that Dr McCallum's evidence was sufficient to provide 'reassurance' to the workers. He agreed with McCallum's conclusion, but added that the study had certain deficiencies and needed following up with a better study.[69]

Dr McCallum had difficulty in funding his continuation of the EMAS study and had to apply for EEC money. Finally, in 1982, 11 years after the EMAS study began, and 9 years after their American equivalents, NIOSH, had completed *their* BCME study (begun at the same time) Dr McCallum completed his preliminary analysis of the EMAS data. He found a significant excess of lung cancer at the Pontyclun plant, which was 20 times the normal rate in the high-exposure group.[70] It is customary to begin scientific articles with a brief review of the evidence to date on the subject being studied. There is no reference to his own negative 1973 study in the review section of Dr McCallum's very positive 1982 draft study.

The saga continues. The GMWU is trying to establish American standards of engineering controls at the Pontyclun plant, and to obtain civil and DHSS compensation for the victims and their families. Since 1979, it has kept the workers up to date with the latest international evidence on BCME, and has tried to expose the whole story with help from the media (BBC Wales did an excellent documentary in 1981). The union has also asked the ombudsman to investigate its charge of maladministration by the Factory Inspectorate and EMAS. No guidance material on the dangers of CME or BCME, nor on the widespread possibility of the accidental formation of BCME by the mixture of formaldehyde and hydrogen chloride, has yet been produced by HSE. The only published reference is in amongst over 500 other substances in the ACGIH list of TLVs published by HSE. A one-line reference towards the back states merely that BCME is a human carcinogen with a TLV of 0.001 ppm, and that CME is also a human carcinogen.

5. Case studies: consumer products

Tobacco

It is generally accepted that over 50,000 people die prematurely in Britain each year, due, at least in part, to cigarette smoking – seven times more than the number who die in road accidents. As the Royal College of Physicians have put it: 'Cigarette smoking is now as important a cause of death as were the great epidemic diseases such as typhoid, cholera and TB that affected previous generations in this country.'[1] In 1979, 34,760 people died from lung cancer in England and Wales and it is estimated that up to 90 per cent of those deaths resulted either directly or indirectly from smoking.[2] Indeed, Britain now has the highest rate of lung cancer in the world, and cigarettes have also been implicated as a major cause of coronary heart disease and chronic bronchitis. Apart from actually killing people, cigarettes also cause much ill-health and suffering, one recent estimate suggesting that smoking-related illness causes the loss of at least 50 million working days in Britain each year.[3] Moreover, the health-damaging effects of smoking extend beyond smokers themselves. Smoking is known to harm those in proximity to smokers, possibly increasing their risks of lung cancer,[4] while mothers who smoke increase the chances of their pregnancy ending in miscarriage, stillbirth or neonatal death;[5] and children of parents who smoke are more likely to suffer from chest infections, bronchitis and pneumonia early in life.[6]

In 1980, about 40 per cent of the adult British population were smokers – 42 per cent of men and 37 per cent of women.[7] This represents a reduction from the 1972 figures (52 per cent and 41 per cent among men and women, respectively), but the rate of decline now seems to have slowed. Indeed, since 1978 there has been evidence of a slight *increase* among unskilled manual workers of both sexes,[8] as well as an increase in the average number of cigarettes consumed.[9] In 1978, only 25 per cent of professional men and 37 per cent of employers and managers were smokers, compared with 53 per cent of semi-skilled and 60 per cent of unskilled workers; these class differences were also found amongst women smokers.[10]

The official explanation for the continuation of such a dangerous habit on a mass scale is that smokers are morally too weak to stop, and therefore have only themselves to blame for the consequences. But, as we have seen, there are at least two important problems with such simple 'victim-blaming'. First, it underestimates the extent to which smoking interacts with other factors to produce its toxic effects: the link between smoking and occupational hazards is especially important here (see appendix 3). Equally fundamentally, it ignores the social and economic pressures which create and maintain the 'need' for cigarettes. In fact, we can only understand the use of nicotine as a dependence-producing drug if we look at the wider social climate which encourages smoking much more strongly than it discourages it.

The enormous advertising and promotion efforts of the tobacco companies misrepresent smoking as desirable, prestigious, and even sexually attractive. Precise figures are difficult to obtain, but recent estimates suggest that in 1980–81 the industry spent some £38 million on newspaper and magazine advertising and £35 million on cinema and poster ads – despite clear evidence that smoking kills people.[11] The response of the tobacco companies to such evidence has not been surprising. In their public utterances at least, they have either tried to cast doubt on the statistical evidence itself,[12] or have claimed that the relationship between smoking and health is something that must be left to 'medical experts'. In the meantime, they have continued the search for a 'safe' cigarette as well as agreeing to place warning signs on packets. (There are, of course, no 'safe' cigarettes and to make up for the missing flavour in low-tar cigarettes, industry adds a wide range of chemicals without labelling them and often without indicating whether they or their inhalant products have been tested for carcinogenicity.) Such palliatives notwithstanding, tobacco companies are committed to maintaining, and if possible expanding, the smoking habit itself, since profits depend on it.

The role of the tobacco companies in promoting smoking is perhaps best illustrated by their present campaign to attract more women smokers. The percentage of smokers in the male population fell substantially from 1961 to 1980, while the proportion of women smokers has hardly changed over the same period,[13] so that the gap between the sexes is narrowing. Moreover, while the cigarette consumption of male smokers rose by about 3 per cent between 1972 and 1980, that of women rose by as much as 15 per cent.[14] Between 1969 and 1978 there was a 50 per cent increase in female lung cancer deaths. In 1980, 8,400 women died from the disease, and the peak of the epidemic has yet to be reached.[15] Indeed, recent estimates suggest that female lung cancer deaths will probably exceed those from breast cancer by the year 2000.

Obviously, there are many factors behind this increase in female smoking, and the changes taking place in women's social and economic roles are an important element in this complex equation. However, it is clear that the activities of the tobacco companies have played a significant part. The 'new woman' was seen to have considerable market potential and the companies switched much of their promotional effort in her direction. Philip Morris spent some £2 million launching their 'liberated' cigarette, Virginia Slims, in 1976, and British America Tobacco followed suit with Kim – the cigarette that is 'long and slender, light and mellow'. Ironically, then, it seems that the apparent 'emancipation' of women may be leading them towards what could be termed the 'diseases of liberation', and that tobacco companies are playing a considerable part in bringing this about.[16]

The capacity of the tobacco industry to continue its deadly activities unabated can be explained partly in terms of its economic and social power. The British cigarette market is at present dominated by three companies. Imperial (through its two companies, Players and Wills) holds about 60 per cent of the market; Gallagher (a subsidiary of the American company American Brands) holds about 27 per cent; and Rothmans International (a multinational company based in Britain but controlled in South

Africa) holds about 13 per cent through its UK company Carreras Rothman.[17] The industry directly employs about 35,000 people in the UK, while a great many others, such as tobacconists and publicans, are heavily dependent on the sale of cigarettes for their livelihood. Moreover, the financially precarious newspaper industry earns more than £30 million each year from cigarette advertising, a fact reflected in the consistent refusal of most newspapers to criticise the industry or to support campaigns for stricter regulation. The power of the industry to control editorial content was starkly revealed in 1980 when W. D. and H. O. Wills threatened to remove £500,000 of advertising revenue from the prestigious *Sunday Times*.[18] The reason was that the paper's medical correspondent, Oliver Gillie, had indicted particular brands of cigarettes in the killing of five men who had been given heart transplants. In the middle of the article was a full-page advertisement for Embassy – one of the cigarettes specifically blamed for helping to kill one of these men. Wills then had the cost of the advertisement in question refunded, and were given another one free. Subsequently, they decided to withdraw £500,000 worth of booked advertising from the paper. Although Wills maintained that this simply reflected a prior decision to switch to the *Sunday Express*, it did result (in January 1981) in the editor of the *Sunday Times*, under pressure from the Board, drafting a statement which he sent to journalists for discussion. If accepted this would have committed the paper to a policy of not campaigning against cigarette advertising. Vigorous objections were made to the statement and it was dropped.[19]

Many sporting events are also dependent on tobacco companies for sponsorship, and this sponsorship is regulated by a 'voluntary agreement' between the industry and the Department of the Environment, in the person of the Minister for Sport. The most recent agreement was reached in March 1982 after protracted negotiations.[20] It allows the companies to spend some £4.5 million per year on sports sponsorship, rising to £6 million by 1985. Industry backing for sporting events has come under strong criticism, first because it is a very efficient way of circumventing other controls on advertising, and, second, because it often reaches young people in particular. Dr Brian Lloyd, Chairman of the Health Education Council, has claimed that the 1982 agreement will lead to some

2,000 extra deaths per year.[21] However, Mr Neil McFarlane, then Minister for Sport, responded by saying that there was 'no conclusive scientific proof' of a link between sponsorship and smoking.[22]

As we have seen, the considerable economic power of the tobacco companies has been important in helping them to escape statutory controls. However, the reasons for the state's failure to control the industry go beyond any concern with the livelihood of those dependent on cigarette manufacturing and sales. Treasury receipts from tobacco tax are now about £4,000 million every year,[23] which means that the state has a direct financial interest in maintaining smoking. Indeed, the Department of Industry actually *subsidises* cigarette manufacturers, having given the industry some £30 million in grants of various kinds since 1972, while the EEC subsidises tobacco farming in France and Italy to the tune of £100 million each year.[24] Thus, government does not oppose but actively supports the tobacco industry. Even more significantly, perhaps, the Ministry of Overseas Development and the Commonwealth Development Corporation have paid three countries (Zambia, Malawi and Belize) at least £3.5 million since 1974 to maintain their tobacco-growing industry – a disturbing example of the increasing use of third world populations as both producers and consumers of tobacco.[25]

It is sometimes argued that the benefits to governments of supporting the tobacco industry may be illusory even when viewed in strictly economic terms. This is because the tax revenue from smokers has to be offset against the cost to the NHS of treating patients with smoking-related diseases – a cost estimated by former Secretary of State for Health David Ennals to be about £2 million *per week* in 1977.[26] Additionally, costs to government include sickness and invalidity benefits, as well as widows' pensions and other death benefits.

But even when these economic calculations are fully accounted, there may still be net savings for the state from tobacco deaths. An item in *New Scientist* reported that:

As a grisly analysis undertaken by the Department of Health three years ago showed, a reduction in cigarette smoking would eventually cost the country more than was gained – not only would there be loss of revenue from taxation but also the additional 'burden' of having to pay out pensions to the people who had given up smoking before it killed them.[27]

Thus, the powerful pressures from the industry, combined with the contradictory and ambivalent position of different government departments, have resulted in failure to develop significant controls over the sale of cigarettes, and no statutory controls have been implemented. Instead, regulation has relied entirely on 'voluntary agreements', and no single department has the responsibility for ensuring their effectiveness. There is ample evidence of the failure of such agreements to curb the promotional activities of the industry, yet no action has been taken against offenders.

Rather than implementing effective controls on the industry, such as banning advertising and imposing heavier taxes, government policies have consisted mainly of moral exhortations to stop smoking. The contradictions inherent in such a policy are highlighted by comparing the £1 million spent annually by the DHSS on publicising the dangers of smoking with the £80 million spent by the industry on spreading the opposite message. This trivial spending on preventive and educational strategies is reinforced by the priorities of the British cancer research organisations. The American Cancer Society has been criticised for failing to take a more aggressive stance against the tobacco industry, and the same criticism can be levelled against the British charities. Indeed, their record is considerably worse, as a recent editorial in the *British Medical Journal* pointed out. While the American Cancer Society is not renowned for its lobbying zeal, it does spend 17 per cent of its funds on educational activities. On the other hand, the British charities – the Cancer Research Campaign and the Imperial Cancer Research Fund – each spend only about 2 per cent of their income on directly educational or preventive projects.[28] Thus, prestige medical projects oriented towards the search for a cure continue to attract a disproportionate share of resources, while the promotional activities of the tobacco industry continue unabated and many thousands die prematurely each year as a result of a largely preventable form of cancer.

Synthetic food colours: the case of amaranth

In 1924, the Departmental Committee on Preservatives and Colouring Matters in Food recommended issuing a list of permitted synthetic food colours. The British government failed to act, and the use of a wide range of these materials persisted in a relatively uncontrolled fashion until the late 1950s. It was only the existence of a growing body of research findings that led to any general policy revision.

In 1936, the dye Butter Yellow, 4-dimethylaminoazobenzene, which had been used extensively in earlier years to colour dairy products and margarine, was shown by Kinosita, a Japanese scientist, to be a very potent carcinogen when fed to rats.[29] One year later, in 1937, Schiller showed that another food colour, Light Green SF, when administered by subcutaneous injection to rats, resulted in sarcomas at the site of injection.[30] In 1949, Kirby and Peacock found that Oil Orange E, another popular commercial dye used in margarine, caused a significantly higher incidence of liver tumours in mice when administered by subcutaneous injection. The authors concluded:

> A commercial dye at present in use for colouring human food in this country had yielded a significant number of liver tumours in mice and seems to justify our contention that synthetic substances of no food value sold for artificially colouring food should be subject to stricter control.[31]

Following these results Oil Orange E was withdrawn from sale.

These experimental findings encouraged the Preservatives Subcommittee of the Food Standards Committee, appointed in 1951, to give early attention to the question of food colours. Its report, published in 1954, included the first recognition by a British expert committee on food additives of the important problem of carcinogenicity testing. Although recognising the difficulties surrounding such testing the committee laid down a general principle: 'Until the contrary can be proved, suspicion must fall on any colour proposed for use in foods which is capable of producing neoplastic reaction in animals.'[32]

This view led the subcommittee to reject the demands of a number of industrial organisations for the continued use of Light Green SF. However, although the subcommittee was prepared to give due weight to any experimental evidence suggesting carcinogenic activity (by whatever method it was demonstrated), it did not adopt such a firm approach towards colours which had simply been insufficiently investigated. A total of 79 colours had been submitted to it as being in use for colouring food at that time. The pharmacology panel, comprising the medical members of the subcommittee, classified the colours under consideration into three categories:

Class A colours which appeared to be innocuous when consumed in the amounts customarily used for colouring foods

Class B colours for which evidence was scanty or conflicting, but for which there was at present no reason to suggest that they were potentially harmful in the amounts ordinarily consumed in foods

Class C colours which have been shown to have, or are suspected to have, harmful effects on health

The subcommittee proposed that in future food colours should be regulated by means of a 'permitted list' which should include not only those in Class A but also those in Class B 'to the extent that the Class A colours are insufficient to meet reasonable trade requirements'. This approach appeared to owe more to expediency in the face of commercial pressures than to the fulfilment of the subcommittee's stated policy that only colours for which there was 'adequate evidence' of safety should be used in foods.

The subcommittee did not object to the use of synthetic colours 'to replace natural colour lost during processing, to standardise appearance or simply to render a product more attractive'. Nevertheless, some scientists held a contrary view. Peacock, who had shown Oil Orange E to be a carcinogen, argued for a much more cautious approach: 'As human life is of more than scientific interest it seems better to err on the side of safety and not to encourage the addition of substances of unpredictable potentiality in human food . . . their addition in order to give a more attractive appearance is not justifiable.'[33]

Even though the Preservatives Subcommittee was pursuing a more accommodating approach than this, its insistence on regulation by a permitted list aroused the opposition of some industrial interests. Eventually, after considerable lobbying and consultation, a permitted list of 29 colours was passed into law in 1957.[34] This was 33 years after such a policy had first been recommended by an official expert advisory body in Britain.

In the period since this first permitted list of colours, there has been considerable controversy over the safety of and need for individual substances included on it. The list has had to be modified and reduced on a number of occasions. One of the permanent members of the permitted list has been the synthetic red colour amaranth.

In 1970, a Russian study was published which concluded that 'chemically pure amaranth possesses carcinogenic activity of medium strength and should not be used in the food industry.'[35] The American Food and Drug Administration subsequently initiated its own carcinogenicity tests on the colour (known in the USA as 'F, D and C Red Dye No. 2') but these were conducted in an unsatisfactory manner with widespread mixing and general neglect of the animals involved. Epstein describes the outcome: 'Enough data were salvaged, however, to demonstrate that at the highest dose, at least, the dye induced a large number of malignant tumors in female rats surviving to two years. That was enough to finally force FDA Commissioner Schmidt to ban the food color in January 1976.'[36]

In Britain, the extensive use of amaranth as a food colour has a long history. By 1923, it had already become one of the six top-sellers in the food-dye market and one major manufacturer was selling over 2.27 tonnes per year.[37] A 1976 survey by the Food Additives and Contaminants Committee showed amaranth to be consumed in a wide variety of food products, including breakfast cereals, canned fruit, canned soup, chocolate, sweets, dessert mixes, ice cream, jellies and preserves. The 'average level of use' was calculated as 1.44mg per day and the 'maximum level of use' as 16.59mg per day.[38]

In its 1954 report, the Food Standards Committee classified amaranth in Class A, which 'are colours which, from the available evidence, would seem unlikely to be harmful when consumed in foods in the customary amounts'. However, the committee also acknowledged that they were 'unable to recommend any colour unreservedly as safe'.[39] A 1964 report again concluded that there was sound evidence of the acceptability of amaranth, even though the full experimental and testing requirements had not been met.[40] As a result of these evaluations, amaranth has been on the British permitted list of food colours since the list was first introduced in 1957.

Following the 1970 Russian studies, which suggested the carcino-genicity of amaranth, the British Industrial Biological Research Association (BIBRA) reviewed the evidence. BIBRA felt that Andrianova's work could not be criticised (as the FDA had suggested) for using material of unreliable specification, but still claimed that 'it seems probable that the tumours attributed to amaranth in this study are those that would normally occur in any group of rats of this age and that the control animals were not observed.'[41] In the light of the earlier carcinogenicity tests, it claimed that there did not appear to be 'any need to re-evaluate the safety-in-use of amaranth'.

The evidence was again reviewed by the Committee on the Toxicity of Chemicals in Food, Consumer Products and the Environment. It concluded that the evidence which had become available on long-term reproduction studies since the previous review 'cast doubt on the status of the colour'. Unlike BIBRA, the committee did criticise Andrianova's study on the grounds that 'the specification of the material used in this study is uncertain'. The committee, however, concluded that 'in view of the uncertainties raised by the results of the mutagenicity studies', it required that 'a well-conducted carcinogenicity study in the rat' be done within five years. Amaranth was downgraded by the committee to Class B, and thus was defined as being 'provisionally acceptable for use in food, but about which further information is necessary'.[42] Nevertheless, amaranth still remains on Britain's permitted list.

The removal of amaranth from the American market has led to its widespread substitution by another red colour Allura Red ('F, D and C Red Dye No. 40'). This colour was approved by the FDA for use in foods in 1971 although its own guidelines that food additives should be tested for carcinogenicity in at least two animal species had not been met.[43]

The Food Additives and Contaminants Committee in its review of the 1973 regulations received industrial representations for the addition of Allura Red AC to the recommended list. The Committee on the Toxicity of Chemicals in Food, Consumer Products and the Environment stated that only one long-term oral feeding study (in the rat) was available and that this was inadequate. It therefore required the results of long-term studies in two species, and classified Allura Red as Class E – colours 'for which the available evidence is inadequate for an opinion to be expressed as to their suitability for use in food'.

The official British response to both food colours is therefore in sharp contrast to that in the USA. This applies both to the retention of amaranth on the permitted list despite recognised uncertainties and inadequacies in scientific data, and conversely to the refusal to add a new colour, Allura Red, before adequate testing had been completed. As a result, it is amaranth which is available in Britain but banned in the USA, whereas Allura Red, which continues to be used in the USA, is not permitted here.

Saccharin

The artificial sweetener saccharin was discovered in 1879 and has been in use since that time. It is a non-calorie substance with a sweetening power 350 times that of sugar. Although it has a long history, the extent of its use has increased markedly in recent years largely due to the growth in the market for low-calorie soft drinks. In Britain, consumption of saccharin more than tripled between the mid-1950s and mid-1970s[44] and there has probably been an even greater expansion of use in the USA. During the 1960s, saccharin was often used in combination with another artificial sweetener, cyclamate, which, although only one-tenth as sweet, lacked the unpleasant after-taste of saccharin. In 1969, cyclamate was banned in the USA and in Britain after the results of feeding studies on rats which showed an increase in bladder tumours following the administration of a cyclamate–saccharin mixture.[45] After the banning of cyclamate, saccharin became the only permitted artificial sweetener and its use escalated. Increasingly, attention was directed to whether saccharin itself was a carcinogen.

In 1972, the Wisconsin Alumni Research Foundation, in a feeding study which examined the effects of saccharin on two generations of rats, found an increased incidence of bladder cancer in second-generation male rats.[46] Following these results, saccharin was removed from the American 'Generally Recognised as Safe' (GRAS) food-additive list, an action which permitted its continued use but allowed a future ban if there was any further doubt about its safety. A study by the FDA, in 1973, resulted in similar findings. In 1977, a Canadian study on a larger number of rats, fed pure saccharin, produced by the Maumee synthesis, at the level of 5 per cent in the diet, confirmed the earlier results.[47] An FDA analysis of these investigations concluded that 'there are now at least three studies which show saccharin to be a urinary bladder carcinogen in the rat.'[48] In addition, a British study in which rats were fed saccharin after their bladders had first been primed by local instillations of low doses of a nitrosamine-type carcinogen had suggested co-carcinogenic activity of saccharin.[49]

In response to the Canadian carcinogenicity study the acting commissioner of the American FDA, Sherwin Gardner, in March 1977 announced his decision 'to end the use of saccharin in our food and beverages'. Although in 1969 Britain had rapidly followed suit after the American ban on cyclamate, the reaction was different in 1977. Newspaper reports boasted that the British authorities were not going to be rushed into a decision, and that 'no unnecessary urgency' was being shown in response to the American view.[50] An official was quoted as saying that there was a need 'to preserve a sense of proportion and no need to panic'.[51] No official evaluation of the scientific evidence on the safety of saccharin was published at the time by the Food Additives and Contaminants Committee (FACC), although it had advised the government on its continued use,[52] but comments in the scientific and medical literature give some impression of British expert opinion.

The Lancet, in an editorial shortly after the FDA ban, expressed scepticism about the evidence on which this action was based.[53] It rested its case on two arguments. First, the epidemiological studies undertaken in Britain by Richard Doll and Bruce Armstrong, at

Oxford University, claim that there is no connection between bladder cancer and saccharin consumption.[54] Second, they claimed that 'many toxicologists in North America as well as in Britain doubt the relevance of feeding studies involving such unrealistically high levels of incorporation of test substances in the diet'. Additional criticism was expressed by *New Scientist* in an editorial which commented that 'rather more impressive is the evidence of the medical demerits of sucrose.' This comparison of the risks and benefits of artificial sweeteners with those of sugar led the writer to conclude that 'their withdrawal on the most dubious of evidence seems particularly foolhardy.'[55] Statements by the nutritionist Professor John Yudkin about the harmful effects of sugar and his view that saccharin was 'very unlikely' to cause cancer in humans, also received wide press coverage.[56] The British scientists Marian Hicks and J. Chowaniec, of Middlesex Hospital Medical School, argued that the absence of restrictive legislation, such as the Delaney Amendment, meant that in Britain it was possible to weigh risks and benefits before making a decision. They concluded that there was a case for saccharin to be retained.[57]

The publication of a Canadian epidemiological study in autumn 1977, which showed a relationship between saccharin consumption and bladder cancer in males,[58] posed a problem for the earlier reliance on evidence from British studies. However, in an editorial, the *Lancet* criticised the study for reporting 'superficial' analyses and for not dealing adequately with confounding factors. It concluded: 'We judge that most readers will find the case against saccharin unimpressive.'[59] The authors of the study responded at length to the points raised, and argued that it should at least be given the same credence as the earlier and more reassuring British studies.[60] Meanwhile, in the USA the FDA came under substantial pressure from industrial interests, politicians and some scientists to modify its stance, despite the fact that the new commissioner, Donald Kennedy, had, in April 1977, confirmed the proposed ban on saccharin in foods, beverages and cosmetics. As in Britain the arguments against a ban were threefold: (a) The failure of most epidemiological studies to show a link between saccharin and cancer; (b) the importance of the assumed benefits of saccharin in reducing sugar consumption; and (c) doubts about the validity of animal testing.

Regarding the epidemiological studies, Epstein argued:

> the quality of these data do not support the claims of safety . . . first, there may be a latency period of decades between exposure and disease . . . second, the success of epidemiology depends on the availability, for comparative studies, of large populations of exposed and unexposed individuals . . . third, epidemiology even under ideal conditions, is unlikely to be able to detect relatively small increases in cancer incidence. Yet, increases of this order could still result in a large number of excess cancer deaths in the US population.[61]

He concluded that in the light of these limitations none of the apparently negative human saccharin studies could be used to give it a clean bill of health for the following reasons. Large-scale use of saccharin had been too recent for a significant excess of saccharin-induced cancers to have appeared in the general population. With regard to diabetic studies the number of cases involved was inadequate to detect any but the grossest increase in cancer incidence, and in addition diabetics were more likely to die at a relatively young age from complications of their disease rather than from cancer. Finally, the focus of the studies on bladder cancer to the exclusion of cancer at other sites was unjustifiable.

As for the claims made for the value of saccharin in the treatment of diabetes, obesity, dental caries and other disorders, Epstein stated that none of them had been backed up by any published studies. He pointed to the fact that the major consumption of saccharin was by the general population rather than by diabetics and the obese, and also that the relatively scant available literature on these benefits cast doubt on the validity of these claims.[62]

The significance of animal studies was referred to the US Office of Technology Assessment (OTA), which in its report of June 1977 concluded:

1 The doses of saccharin used in the rat cancer tests
  were admittedly high, but were valid.
2 The most convincing animal cancer tests indicate
  that saccharin is a weak carcinogen in rats.

3 Saccharin is also likely to be a relatively weak
   carcinogen in people.
4 Though weak, for several important reasons
   saccharin should be regarded as having the potential
   of posing a significant health hazard to humans.[63]

In spite of arguments such as these, the American Congress
passed legislation in the autumn of 1977 to suspend the FDA ban on
saccharin for 18 months. In March 1978, the Commission of the
European Economic Community recommended that member
states should observe certain provisions concerning saccharin:

1 Regulations should be devised to keep the daily
   intake of saccharin below 2.5mg/kg.
2 The use of saccharin in infant food should be
   prohibited.
3 Foodstuffs should be specifically labelled as
   containing saccharin.
4 Saccharin tablets should be labelled to inform
   the purchaser of the possible dangers of
   excessive consumption of saccharin, especially
   in the case of pregnant women and children.[64]

In response, the Food Additives and Contaminants Committee
(FACC) considered that there was 'no immediate need to recommend
additional restrictions on the use of saccharin in the UK'.[65] No
cautionary labelling was therefore adopted. At the same time, it was
announced that the Committee on Toxicity of Chemicals in Food,
Consumer Products and the Environment (COT) was to undertake
a full evaluation of the safety of saccharin and that FACC would
await the results of this review before advising whether any action
was necessary. It is apparent, therefore, that the British authorities
did not see any urgent need to control saccharin more rigorously
after the findings of carcinogenicity in animals.

In March 1979, a British expert on experimental carcinogenesis,
Eric Boyland, reviewed the animal studies on saccharin, and
concluded that the evidence indicated that saccharin 'may be
considered a weak bladder carcinogen'.[66] He felt that these results
were best explained by seeing saccharin as a promoter of cancer
rather than as carcinogen proper – although this did not necessarily

mean that it was any less dangerous. However, his own view was that 'saccharin is unlikely to provide a serious hazard because the dose required to produce the promoting effect is so large.' In conclusion, he argued that 'the very low, though finite risks may be worth the benefits of its use' – though he did not specify what he thought those benefits might be. In 1982, four years after the beginning of their investigations, FACC and COT published the British assessment of the safety and usefulness of saccharin.[67]

COT concluded that:

> saccharin is associated with an increased incidence of urinary bladder tumours in second generation rats following continuous oral administration at very high doses relative to the amounts consumed by man. However, epidemiological studies have failed to show an association between saccharin use and urinary bladder cancer in man; this is consistent with saccharin being neither a complete carcinogen nor a bladder tumour promoter in humans.

This attempt to use the epidemiological data as a counterweight to the evidence of carcinogenicity in animals should be assessed in the light of two major areas of ignorance acknowledged by the committee: '(a) the mechanism by which saccharin at very high doses, causes bladder tumours in second generation rats *is not known* . . . (b) it is *not known* whether the mechanism(s) that operate(s) in rats would operate in man under conditions of normal dosages, under conditions of very high dosages or when exposure begins *in utero*.'[68]

COT recommended, 'as a measure of prudence', only 'temporary acceptance' of saccharin for use in food. Given that any food additive can be removed from a permitted list in the light of adverse scientific evidence, it is difficult to assess what this 'measure of prudence' amounts to in practice.

FACC recommended that saccharin should remain on the permitted list (along with two new intense sweeteners, acesulfame potassium and aspartame) and reaffirmed its rejection of the EEC recommendation for warning labels on saccharin tablets. In view of the extensive claims for health benefits of saccharin in discouraging sugar consumption which, as we have seen, led a number of experts to consider that these outweighed the risks, it is astonishing that this issue is not seriously treated by the committee. No scientific evidence for the supposed health benefits of widespread usage of saccharin is considered at all. Instead, FACC lists as examples of the 'need' for saccharin: making the 'mouthfeel' of soft drinks more acceptable; making water ices less sticky, and reducing their tendency to surface crystallisation; aiding the freezing of foods; maintaining the 'cloudy' nature of certain concentrated soft drinks; diabetic foods; 'sugar-free' foods; and 'slimming foods'. While these last three 'needs' imply a positive effect on health this is neither evaluated on the basis of any evidence, nor discussed in terms of whether saccharin needs to be generally available in order to achieve it.

Instead, the case for saccharin is summarised by FACC as follows:

> Saccharin has a long history of use in food. Its organoleptic properties in individual food formulations produced on a full commercial scale are well understood and industry regards it of high importance. We accept that there is a continuing and established need for saccharin.[69]

The British system of regulation has often been heralded as superior to the American in one respect: it allows control to be based on a comparative assessment of the benefits against the risks of a food additive. In this case, however, the health benefits of saccharin have simply been stated; no respectable scientific case has been made for them. Instead, a commercial concept of 'need' is paramount, and the toxicological assessment rests on a down-grading of the significance of positive carcinogenic results in animal tests.

Nitrosamines and the food additive nitrite

Nitrosamines are chemicals with a terminal N-nitroso, N-N=O, group. There are a large number of them, many of which are to be found throughout the environment. Most of them have been shown to be highly carcinogenic to a wide range of organs in all animal species tested.[70] About 130 different nitrosamines have been tested, and about 80 per cent shown to be carcinogenic. Carcinogenic properties of nitrosamines have been well established since the 1950s. Nitrosamines can be readily formed in the environment and in the body by the reaction of two types of very common chemical substances – amines and nitrites or nitrogen oxides.[71] It has been suggested by Epstein that nitrosamines and other N-nitroso compounds may be a major class of universal carcinogens responsible for a substantial number of human cancers under a wide range of conditions and circumstances.[72] Although nitrosamines are ubiquitous environmental carcinogens, this study explores the problems arising from just one particular source – the use of nitrites as curing and preserving agents in food.

Research undertaken by the British Food Manufacturers' Research Association (BFMRA) in the late 1920s and 1930s pointed towards the value of nitrites in the curing and preserving of meat products. Since the 1925 Public Health (Preservatives, etc. in Food) Regulations did not explicitly permit their use as preservatives, this posed a problem for the food manufacturers.[73] The BFMRA suggested that 'small quantities of them might not be considered as infringing the Regulations,' but went on to add that 'even if they might be considered as infringing the Regulations it was thought that it might be possible to have the Regulations extended in this direction if they proved valuable from this point of view.'[74] In 1929, BFMRA 'strongly recommended that sodium and potassium nitrite should be used in all curing brines in place of saltpetre,'[75] and added that New Zealand meat packers were being undersold by American packers who used this process because of 'the economies resulting from the use of nitrite'.[76] In the late 1930s, the Preservatives Regulations were amended so as to permit the use of nitrites in curing meats, but with certain limitations – cooked meats were not permitted to contain more than 200 ppm at the time of sale. No limits were fixed by these regulations for nitrite in bacon and hams, but a licence was required for the process from the Bacon Control Department of the Ministry of Food.[77] This requirement was later abandoned under the Bacon Revocation Order of 1954.

The Preservatives Subcommittee of the Food Standards Committee considered the use of nitrate and nitrite in 1959 and 1960. Although it stated that a limit on the nitrite and nitrate content of bacon and ham was desirable, it was unable to specify any particular limit because there was insufficient evidence about the existing levels of nitrate and nitrite at point of retail sale.[78] The subsequent Preservatives in Food Regulations of 1962,[79] made under the Food and Drugs Act (1955) permitted the use of nitrates in bacon, ham and pickled meats without limit, and in some cheeses up to 100 ppm. Nitrites were allowed in bacon and ham without limit, in cooked pickled meats up to 200 ppm; in uncooked pickled meats up to 500 ppm and in certain cheeses up to 10 ppm.

It was suggested as early as 1963 that nitrites and secondary amines present in food could react with each other in the acidic environment of the stomach to form nitrosamines.[80] However, it was the identification of dimethylnitrosamine in fish meal preserved with sodium nitrite in Norway that initially aroused the concern of the British regulatory authorities.[81] When the renamed BFMRA – now the British Food Manufacturing Industries Research Association (BFMIRA) – learned of these findings, members were extremely disturbed and the director of research, C. L. Cutting, circulated an anxious letter to its members in the meat industry.[82] The letter stated:

It is known to the Research Association that there is concern in official circles over the possible occurrence in cured meat products of nitrosamine formed by the action of nitrites added or formed during the curing process on minor components of the meat. These compounds are known to be powerful cancer-producing agents in a wide range of animals and there appears to be a danger that the whole process of curing may be called in question. The Research Association has already mounted a limited attempt to establish by direct analysis whether or not nitrosamines are present in commercial cured meat products. Using published methods, indications of the presence of nitrosamines have been obtained but it has become clear that the problem cannot be satisfactorily resolved on this limited basis. *Certainly the RA has at the moment no evidence to satisfy the authorities in the event of a challenge on this aspect of the safety of nitrite use.* In view of the grave potential importance of this issue to the meat-curing industry it is felt to be urgently necessary to increase the effort of the RA in this direction.[83]

It is apparent, then, that BFMIRA were defining the problem primarily as one of establishing the presence of nitrosamines in food products, without contesting the potency of nitrosamines as carcinogens.

It had, of course, been work by British scientists which had shown that, in rats, an 'outstanding characteristic' of nitrosamines was that they could be 'one-shot' carcinogens (i.e. a single exposure could ultimately lead to tumours).[84] An editorial in the *Lancet* in May 1968 emphasised that the presence of nitrosamines in food was 'a matter of the gravest concern' and acknowledged that they could be formed by the interaction of nitrites with amines present in food. It went on to add, however, that 'any possible risk to human health arising from the addition of nitrites to food must be balanced against their value as preservatives, especially their action against Clostridia.'[85]

In October 1968, a joint meeting was held between the Pharmacology Subcommittee, FACC and the BFMIRA to define a programme of research on nitrosamines,[86] which included 'dose-response' studies at low levels of nitrosamine exposure. These were subsequently initiated. In 1970, workers at the Courtauld Institute reported that *in vitro* metabolism of dimethylnitrosamine in humans and rats were very similar. They went on to suggest that

man may be about as sensitive as the rat to the carcinogenic action of this compound. In view of the high carcinogenicity of the nitrosamines and their presence in the environment, our findings emphasise the potential human hazard from exposure to this group of carcinogens.[87]

In February 1971, FACC made an interim report recommending that 'as a first step, limits should be imposed on the nitrate and nitrite content of bacon, ham and pickled meats'.[88] These recommendations were implemented in new regulations passed in 1971, limiting the level of nitrate to 500 ppm and nitrite to 200 ppm.[89]

A review of the situation was undertaken by the Pharmacology Subcommittee of FACC in July 1971; this resulted in the classification of nitrites and nitrates as 'provisionally acceptable' pending 'resolution of the nitrosamine problem', and subject to the results of long-term studies on mice and dogs given sodium nitrite in their diet.[90] FACC's review in 1972 referred to studies on the presence of nitrosamines in various foods, but observed that the amounts of nitrosamines so far detected were minute and far below the levels at which such substances had been biologically tested. It felt that no other restrictions were required at that time, and while calling on the industry to take steps as soon as possible to reduce the use of nitrate and nitrite, and to examine the feasibility of the total elimination of one or both of these substances, the aim of the research programme that had been initiated was defined as studying the 'exact levels required'. It stated that the limits should be reconsidered within two years.[91]

An editorial in the *Lancet* the following year claimed that the relevance of existing studies to human cancer was 'difficult to judge', and that there was 'no direct evidence that man is susceptible'. It was considered unwise to assume that humans were resistant to nitrosamine carcinogens, but the gap identified in the evidence was that there were no experimental data available on dose–response curves at very low levels. These were felt to pose 'formidable technical problems'.[92] It is apparent, then, that during the preceding five years the problem had been redefined by industry and government from a major issue requiring action to one of a long-term research programme to explore dose–response relationships at low levels.

In 1976, the Laboratory of the Government Chemist published a survey of the levels of nitrosamine in over 500 foods in Britain. They were identified in a number of meat, bacon, fish and cheese products. The report saw its task as ensuring that the concentrations present in food were below a level which was hazardous to humans, and it referred to other studies whose aim was 'to identify, if possible, guidelines for maximum permitted levels'.[93] This growing preoccupation with identification of a 'safe level' was the background to the low-key British response to the nitrosamine problem.

In the USA, on the other hand, the established presence of nitrosamines in bacon led the Department of Agriculture (USDA), in May 1978, to set a new limit of 120 ppm for nitrite, and a maximum level for nitrosamine formation of 10 parts per billion (ppb) in bacon.[94] In the summer of 1978, the questions surrounding the use of nitrite in food were confusingly broadened by a report from Paul Newberne of the Massachusetts Institute of Technology (MIT) that nitrite itself might be carcinogenic. Up until this point, the concern had been primarily with the carcinogenic risks of nitrosamine formation, whether formed exogenously (e.g. in food) or endogenously (i.e. in the human body). Newberne reported that rats who had been fed nitrite had an increased incidence of cancers of the lymphatic system.[95] Following this report, the FDA announced, in 1978, its intention gradually to eliminate the use of nitrite in food.[96] During 1979 and 1980, however, the Newberne study was reviewed by a group of non-government pathologists, as well as by the FDA and USDA. This led the regulatory agencies to state that there was 'insufficient evidence' to support the conclusion that nitrite had directly induced cancer in the rats, and, in August 1980, the proposed elimination was abandoned.[97] No regulatory action was considered necessary in Britain during this period and MAFF simply referred data to its expert committees for evaluation and advice.[98]

Meanwhile, further work on the nitrosamine problem was being completed in Britain. A study sponsored by MAFF had been initiated in 1972 at BIBRA and completed by 1978. No results of this study have yet been published in Britain, but there have been references to them by an FDA official[99] and an American journalist.[100] These commentators stated that the findings of the study were that in rats dimethylnitrosamine at the very lowest dose level tested (33 ppb) still produced hyperplastic liver nodules (a precancerous condition) and at 132 ppb produced liver cancer. Statistical analyses of the data have been undertaken by BIBRA and Richard Peto, but no government assessment of the findings had emerged by March 1981, nearly a year after the American press reports of this British government-sponsored study. This has been described as a 'glacial pace' by an American observer who described the British situation as follows:

The British government can sit on a government-sponsored study as long as it chooses. Britain has no Freedom of Information Act, but it does have a government secrets and confidentiality act that permits it to withhold scientific data from the public.[101]

The response of a British government official to this view was: 'The Act may stifle lively scientific exchanges but it also prevents a "Newberne-type fiasco".'[102]

Female sex hormones*

A wide variety of female sex hormones is available for use and they are often referred to in different ways. In order to avoid confusion we therefore begin with a summary of the different types.

Female sex hormones can be divided into two major categories, oestrogens and progestogens (or progestins). In the body, there are three naturally occurring oestrogens – oestradiol, oestriol and oestrone – and one progestogen, called progesterone. In addition to the oestrogens mentioned above, others used in therapy or in animal feed are either derived from pregnant mares' urine (hence 'premarin' – sometimes termed natural since it comes from an animal), or are manufactured synthetically (like ethinyl oestradiol, mestranol or diethylstilboestrol). Synthetic progestogens include substances like medroxyprogesterone acetate (Depo Provera), norgestrel and norethisterone. Progesterone itself is rarely used therapeutically since it is not active when taken orally, but only by injection or suppository.

In Britain, large numbers of women have been or are currently exposed to extra oestrogens and progestogens. Over 3 million women now take oral contraceptive pills,[103] while around a quarter of a million are on hormone replacement therapy.[104] Approximately 7,500 pregnant women are known to have been treated with diethylstilboestrol (DES) between 1940 and 1971 – mostly during the 1950s – and other unspecified oestrogens were given to a further 4,500 pregnant women, mainly during the 1960s.[105] In addition, there is an unknown level of exposure to sex hormone residues in meat from permitted feed additives and implants used to promote growth. These include DES and derivatives of the male hormone, testosterone. While the Ministry of Agriculture claims that residues in British meat have always been lower here than in the USA, it is worth noting the recent scandals in France and Italy involving

---

* This section was contributed by Sue Barlow and Jill Rakusen.

illegally injected veal.[106] In 1979, for example, 12 per cent of French veal was condemned because of 'over use' of artificial hormones.[107]

Hormones in pregnancy

The prescription of DES to pregnant women some decades ago provides one of the most disturbing examples of iatrogenic disease in general, and hormone-induced cancer in particular. Prescription of DES began in the 1950s, supposedly to prevent threatened abortion or premature labour. Only in 1971,[108] after thousands of women had been exposed, particularly in the USA, was it discovered that the drug had a tragic, late-developing effect on some of the daughters of the pregnant women concerned. As teenagers, or young women, some of these 'DES' daughters developed a rare cancer of the vagina. Many of the others, on examination, were observed to have 'vaginal adenosis'[109] – a little-understood cell abnormality which may or may not result in cancer at some stage in the future.[110] In addition, many of the women exposed *in utero* were found to have other abnormalities of the reproductive organs or genitalia, such as irregularly shaped uteri.[111]

We still do not know the full extent of the damage caused by the prescription of this drug during pregnancy. Recent reports indicate that 'DES' daughters have more difficulties carrying a healthy pregnancy to term,[112] that male offspring suffer from damage to their reproductive organs,[113] and that the mothers who themselves were given the drug may be at an increased risk of breast cancer.[114] To make matters worse, research in the 1950s showed that the drug was ineffective.[115] Indeed, when this research was re-examined over 20 years later, it was found that DES had in fact increased the incidence of miscarriage and baby deaths.[116]

The DES story serves as a clear warning to any doctor willing to consider prescribing hormones to pregnant women, but by no means all of them have learnt from this tragedy. Other hormones are still commonly prescribed during pregnancy (though not so much in Britain) despite there being no proof of their safety or efficacy, and the existence of long-standing evidence linking them with congenital malformations.[117] In some countries, 30–40 per cent of pregnant woman are given these drugs in an attempt to avert the same problems that DES failed to help.[118]

Oral contraceptives

There is widespread use in Britain of the 'combined' oral contraceptive (i.e. containing both oestrogen and progestogen). 'Sequential' pills (two weeks on oestrogen, one week on oestrogen and progestogen, one week off) have now been taken off the market. It is interesting, however, that this decision was taken because of their relatively low efficacy in preventing pregnancy, rather than because of what was known about their association with an increased risk of cancer.[119] As for the constituents of the combined pills, there is ample evidence from animal studies that many of the oestrogens and progestogens used are carcinogenic when given in high doses, and occasionally – with oestrogens – even in low doses.[120]

It is not surprising that sex hormones in high doses should cause cancer in animals, since the physiological actions of naturally occurring sex hormones in the body do include stimulating the growth of reproductive tissues. Most other carcinogens interfere at the genetic level to cause changes in the chromosomes which results in disordered growth. This means that a single genetic event may be sufficient to cause cancer, and, also, that there is no 'threshold' exposure below which a carcinogen may be considered safe. However, because of the normal stimulatory mechanism of action of sex hormones, there *may* be a dose below which they are relatively safe. One proviso, though, is that oestrogen and progestogen should be given together, since progestogen has an inhibitory action on oestrogen's stimulatory effects. The relevance of this to carcinogenicity is not, however, clear.

Although at the moment the risk of cancer from oral contraceptive use seems small, it is not yet possible to estimate the true risk because of the latency period that can exist between exposure to carcinogens and the appearance of cancer. Nevertheless, it is clear that oral contraceptives can cause liver tumours, and both the benign and malignant forms can be fatal. To date, 257 cases of liver tumours associated with pill usage have been reported worldwide.[121] Cervical cancer appears to be no higher in pill users than in Intra-Uterine Device (IUD) users,[122] but some women with cervical dysplasia before starting on the Pill may be at increased risk of developing cervical cancer.[123] It remains to be seen whether long-term exposure to the Pill during reproductive years may increase the risks of uterine, breast or other cancers in later life.

Injectable contraceptives

In recent years, there has been considerable controversy over the use of medroxyprogesterone acetate (Depo Provera, or DP) as an injectable contraceptive. Each injection lasts upwards of three months. It is currently licensed in Britain for short-term use only, either by women who have had a rubella vaccination or whose partners have just been vasectomised and who need protection until the sperm count drops to zero. However, it is now recognised that DP is being used much more widely and on a long-term basis, particularly amongst women who may be least able to understand the possible risks and side-effects, and who may not even be informed of them.[124] It is estimated that, in 1978, 33,000 women received DP in this country,[125] and it is being used particularly in areas of social deprivation and among Black and Asian women.

Apart from the known side-effects of this drug, which include severe menstrual disruption, ranging across continuous and/or heavy bleeding, spotting, and complete suppression of periods, there is also strong evidence that it is a carcinogen in animals. When tested in beagles, it has resulted in malignant breast tumours, and in monkeys has caused uterine cancer.[126] Although the drug has been in widespread use among women in over 70 countries, it has mostly been administered as part of population control programmes, and no groups of women have yet been systematically followed up to assess the cancer or other long-term risks. In the light of the carcinogenicity tests in beagles, the FDA banned the use of DP as a contraceptive in the USA. For some time, the British Committee on Safety of Medicines (CSM) had refused to extend the licence for DP to long-term use, but recently changed their minds, recommending that it should be licensed for long-term use. Although reasons for this change were not given, it implies that the committee no longer thought the animal species and/or the doses of DP used for testing were relevant to the human situation. Whilst the beagle may well have unique responses to progestogens, there is little evidence to suggest that the monkey also has idiosyncratic reactions to DP. The UK Minister of Health has, however, refused to accept the recommendation of the CSM (as of December 1982) – though out of concern about its use in the mentally handicapped, rather than doubt about the cancer risks.[127]

Although a licence has not been granted, any doctor in this country can prescribe any drug for indications and lengths of time other than those for which it is licensed. Furthermore, another injectable contraceptive, norethisterone oenanthate, has now been licensed for short-term use by the CSM. Less is known about this drug than about DP, but animal tests suggest that it may be a carcinogen and it is also of lower contraceptive efficacy than DP.[128]

Hormone-replacement therapy (HRT)

In women, the increased risk of uterine cancer from HRT when given as oestrogen alone is well established.[129] In other sites – ovary and breast, for example – the connection between HRT and cancer is, as yet, less well documented.

The British reaction to HRT has been substantially different from that of the USA, where it is freely prescribed and sometimes for very long periods. In Britain, doctors have often refused HRT even in those severe cases of menopausal problems in which it might possibly be indicated. Moreover, such menopause clinics as do exist should be viewed with some suspicion, since most of the research conducted in them is funded by the drug firms supplying the HRT, and a relationship of this kind between clinician, patient and financier scarcely makes for an objective assessment of the drug in question. On the other hand, many GPs who are prepared to prescribe HRT are often totally ignorant of the screening and monitoring that are essential to its use, and unaware of the need to use the lowest possible dose for the shortest possible time. Unlike women in the USA, women in Britain are not given written information about HRT in the form of a drug package insert.

A further major difference between the two countries has been the development in Britain of a combined oestrogen–progestogen HRT. Recent indirect evidence from biopsies suggests that perhaps the way oestrogen is administered may alter its carcinogenic potential. If it is given cyclically and with added progestogen, the risk of uterine cancer – estimated to be increased several-fold in the American studies where oestrogen alone was given – may be reduced.[130] Although this work has been pioneered in Britain, very few prescriptions have been given for this combined therapy, and no satisfactory epidemiological studies on women using it are yet available. Limited epidemiological evidence from the USA suggests that cyclic use alone does not protect against endometrial cancer, but that addition of a progestogen may provide partial protection.[131]

Finally, while Premarin still remains one of the most widely used HRT drugs in this country, it should be noted that the American studies of uterine cancer and HRT did not implicate Premarin alone, and HRT involving other synthetic oestrogens also appeared to increase the incidence of uterine cancer.[132]

Occupational hazards

Oestrogens are manufactured in Britain, and problems similar to those encountered in the USA[133] have also been found among British workers. In one factory (Thomas Kerfoot of Ashton-under-Lyme) the workforce was restricted to post-menopausal women after the development of enlarged breasts in a male worker and increased bloodclotting in younger women workers. (There is, however, no evidence that it is any safer to expose older women to oestrogens.)

Conclusion

Despite the widespread use of sex hormones for many different reasons over many years, we are still not in a position to assess their true risks. Indeed, there can be no doubt that, despite a certain amount of prior animal testing, it is women who have been – and are still being – used as guinea pigs in assessing the risks of the Pill and all other sex hormones.

6. Case studies:
the general environment

Chlorinated hydrocarbon pesticides

Aldrin and the closely related dieldrin (referred to here as A/D) and chlordane and heptachlor (referred to here as C/H) are highly persistent organochlorine insecticides used in large quantities in Britain and the USA from the 1950s to the 1970s. A/D is manufactured exclusively in Britain and in the USA by Shell, the Anglo-Dutch company; C/H is made by the American company, Velsicol. The history of the regulation of A/D and C/H provides an object lesson on the theme of this book – namely, that political and economic factors exert a crucial influence on decisions about what causes cancer and how carcinogens should be controlled.

Aldrin and dieldrin
It was first suggested that A/D might be carcinogenic in 1962 when the US Food and Drug Administration (FDA) published a study which showed liver cancers in mice fed with 10 ppm A/D.[1] A US Health Department commission (the 'Mrak Commission') reported in 1969 that A/D should be considered carcinogenic substances. In 1971, the newly formed Environment Protection Agency (EPA), under pressure from various environmentalist groups, proposed severe restrictions on the use of these pesticides. The proposal that A/D be, in effect, banned was based on the application of the so-called 'nine cancer principles', the last of which states that 'any substance which produces tumors in animals must be considered a carcinogenic hazard in man if the results are achieved according to the established parameters of a valid carcinogenesis test.'[2]

The EPA's proposal – and the nine principles themselves – were challenged by Shell in public hearings that lasted 1,700 days. In particular, Shell, and the consultants they called in defence of A/D, challenged the use of the mouse as the 'test animal' for proof of carcinogenicity. They also argued that animal tests in general should be discounted, whatever their findings, since epidemiological studies of workers exposed to high levels of A/D had supposedly shown no excess of cancers.

Despite the long and apparently technical arguments, the hearings can be seen as a conflict between two philosophies of carcinogen control. One argues that epidemiological evidence should be given priority – that is, that evidence for a substance's supposed carcinogenicity should be sought in the medical records of those workers who can be shown to have been exposed to the substance. The other philosophy sees evidence from valid well designed animal experiments as taking priority over epidemiological data, especially if the latter are inadequate. Although no animal can be an exact analogue for human exposure, if a significant incidence of cancers are induced by the suspected carcinogen then this is deemed sufficient evidence *for regulatory purposes*, especially if the tests are replicated in different strains and species of test animals, to strongly control or even ban the suspected carcinogen. The first philosophy is thus a retrospective approach, which gives a substance the benefit of the doubt, while the second is a more prospective, cautious approach.

In this particular case, the 'animal data' philosophy eventually won out. In 1976, A/D was banned in the USA on the grounds of imminent carcinogenic hazard. The ban, explains Epstein, was due to:

> the combined efforts of a public interest group and the EPA's Office of General Counsel aided by a small team of independent experts. These were pitted against the massive legal and scientific resources of Shell and the US Department of Agriculture, which supported Shell's position, aided by the politically powerful Southern Congressional network and its own Office of Pesticide Programs, which was hostile to the proceedings.[3]

In Britain, evidence of the carcinogenicity of A/D has been considered on three occasions by the Pesticide Safety Precautions Schemes (PSPS) Advisory Committee, the ACP (in 1964, 1969 and 1974), and once by the Food Additives and Contaminants Committee (FACC), in 1967. The earlier committees, in 1964 and 1967, merely requested more data to clarify the issue, but the later committees claimed A/D *not* to be carcinogenic. The 1969 committee, reviewing the 1962 American FDA experiments, which showed the induction of liver tumours in mice by A/D, could reach no consensus as to whether the tumours were 'benign' or 'malignant'. The committee also hinted that their induction might be unique to the mouse −a position similar to that asserted by Shell in the American regulatory hearings. The 1969 committee report placed great stress on the supposedly negative epidemiological evidence derived from Dutch studies of Shell workers.[4] Indeed, the committee considered that animal experiments could only provide presumptive evidence and that, in the light of the lack of human confirmation, A/D could continue to be used.

In October 1974, after the suspension hearings and the decision to ban A/D in the USA, a medical panel of the PSPS met and reported that 'there was no reason to recommend any change in the UK action on aldrin and dieldrin as decided at the time of the 1969 Review of Organochlorine Pesticides.'[5] It seems, therefore, that the general insistence by Shell on the need for excessively rigid criteria of carcinogenicity has been accepted in Britain. This is illustrated by the willingness of the British committee to accept Shell's epidemiological evidence − however flawed − and their implicit rejection of animal carcinogenicity data which had already been accepted by the EPA and many eminent scientists. The medical profession in Britain, as reflected in the *Lancet* and the *British Medical Journal*,[6] also appears to have accepted the epidemiological evidence and was generally 'anti-EPA'.

It is difficult to escape the view that, although much of the debate was couched in technical and scientific terms, the crucial factor in these decisions was the belief in the economic importance of A/D to British agriculture. PSPS committees were well aware of the agricultural industry's views as to the cost that would be incurred − in crop losses, for instance − if A/D were banned or severely restricted. However, this information was not made public, so that there was no opportunity for independent assessment or for alternative views (e.g. about the cancer risk to consumers, or about evidence from the USA on the ineffectiveness of A/D) to be put. The 1969 PSPS report did in fact express concern at the disappointingly slow development of alternative and less persistent control methods. It recommended that studies be undertaken to ascertain the extra cost to industry to safety testing, and to estimate what measures could be taken to stimulate the innovation of environmentally rational control techniques. However, no such report has been made public and the situation changed little until January 1981 when an EEC Directive meant that in theory at least, the use of aldrin had to be restricted to only three specified circumstances, though in practice its use continues to be widespread.

Chlordane and heptachlor

In 1969, the Mrak Commission, on the basis of an FDA mouse study, concluded that heptachlor was carcinogenic.[7] However, since two unpublished reports commissioned by Velsicol had come to the opposite conclusion, it was not until November 1974 that the EPA announced that it intended to seek a ban on the use of C/H in line with the ban on A/D. In the three years of hearings and litigation that followed, Velsicol opposed the EPA proposal in a similar manner to Shell's opposition to the banning of A/D – that is, they attacked the 'nine cancer principles' as a dubious basis for the regulation of pesticides. Finally, it was agreed only to phase out all agricultural uses of C/H over a five-year period, and to continue to allow its use for termite control; such use is coming under increasing challenge in the USA, largely because of growing evidence of the frequency of contamination of homes following termite treatment.

In Britain, the use of C/H had already been severely restricted on environmental grounds since 1964 – long before pressure ever arose to consider its carcinogenicity. This decision was taken after great pressure from ornithological groups concerned both about the large number of bird deaths associated with the use of C/H, and about problems of persistence. There does not seem to have been great resistance by farmers to the restriction, and, despite decisions in 1969 and 1974 to restrict further the approved uses of C/H, MAFF now claims that virtually all agricultural use had ceased by 1967. Thus, it seems that in the UK there has never been any official consideration of the carcinogenicity of C/H.

The ease of this restriction, compared to the massive resistance of American agricultural interests to the banning of C/H, can be explained by the relatively low economic importance of C/H in the UK. In 1964, the crops on which they were used – mainly sugar beet and wheat – could equally well be protected by alternative pesticides, especially A/D. Indeed, the 1964 report recommending restriction of C/H specifically recognised that A/D could be used instead. It emphasised the great importance of A/D to British crop protection and the massive losses that would occur if their use was restricted. There was little or no resistance by industrial interests to C/H restriction, which may be explained by the fact that their main international manufacturer was an American firm (Velsicol) whilst A/D was made by a half-British concern (Shell).

The virtual banning of C/H in Britain and the lack of any other 'economically viable' alternative to A/D greatly increased the use of the latter in British agriculture. Conversely, in the USA, the suspension of A/D increased the use of C/H as an alternative. C/H had always been of greater economic importance in the USA than in Britain because of their effectiveness against the pests of major crops such as cotton, corn, wheat, citrus fruits, tobacco – the banning of A/D made them even more important.

2,4,5-Trichlorophenoxyacetic acid (2,4,5-T)

The herbicide (weed-killer) 2,4,5-T has become the focus of a major controversy in Britain, the repercussions of which may well alter the whole future pattern of pesticide regulation. A vigorous campaign to ban its use has recently been mounted by various trade unions, with the support of the TUC General Council and the Labour Party.[8]

2,4,5-T is a plant-hormone analogue that kills by artificially stimulating growth, so that plants collapse and die under their own excessive weight. It is manufactured in a series of chemical reactions from trichlorophenol during one of which a highly persistent and toxic impurity is formed – TCDD (2,3,7,8-tetrachlorodibenzo-p-dioxin – frequently referred to simply as 'dioxin'). TCDD is one of the most toxic synthetic organic chemicals known and one of the most potent known carcinogens and teratogens (i.e. substance causing birth defects). It can induce cancers and injure or kill embryos at doses lower than one-billionth of a gram per kilogram of body weight per day.[9]

2,4,5-T has been produced since the 1940s, and first came to public attention during the Vietnam war when American planes sprayed some 11 million gallons of 'Agent Orange' as a defoliant. The major ingredients of 'Agent Orange' were 2,4,5-T and the related herbicide 2,4-dichlorophenoxyacetic acid (2,4-D). The consequences of this action have provided additional human evidence on the toxicity of 2,4,5-T. Examination of South Vietnamese refugees and North Vietnamese exposed to the herbicide have shown suggestive evidence of an increased incidence of various clinical abnormalities, including birth deformities, miscarriages and sterility.[10] American troops were also exposed to 2,4,5-T, both directly (by inhalation) and indirectly (by contamination of water and food), and the manufacturers at present face a series of 'class action suits' on behalf of a number of Vietnam veterans for sums in the region of 40 billion dollars.

In addition to studies based on exposure in Vietnam, reports have also emerged in recent years based on occupational accidents and occupational exposures in various contexts. Many of these reports have pointed to the existence of toxic effects similar to those found in experimental animals and in troops in Vietnam. The contaminant TCDD has been linked to a wide range of acute and delayed effects, including a persistent and disfiguring skin disease (known as chloracne), muscular weakness, pains in limbs and joints, nausea and digestive tract disturbances, abnormalities in liver function, increase in blood lipids, porphyria, peripheral neuropathy, and behavioural abnormalities. On the specific question of carcinogenic effects, epidemiological evidence of excess rates of cancers, especially the very rare and lethal soft tissue sarcomas, comes in particular from a number of recent Swedish studies on occupationally exposed workers; soft tissue sarcomas have been reported in Vietnam veterans, workers occupationally exposed to TCDD, and in women living in Midland County, Michigan, in proximity to the Dow Chemical plant which had been manufacturing 2,4,5-T for over three decades.[11] In addition to TCDD exposure via direct means, such as inhalation and skin contact, the possible concentration and accumulation of TCDD in human and animal body fats must also be considered.[12] In view of the very high toxicity and carcinogenicity of TCDD, any such concentrations could be extremely injurious to health.

It is evidence of this kind, and, in particular, the strong evidence that 2,4,5-T is teratogenic, that has led a number of countries to ban the use of 2,4,5-T. At present, these include Italy, Holland, Sweden, Denmark, Japan and the USA (for forestry, rights-of-way and pasture use). In Britain, the efficacy and safety of pesticides is under the control of MAFF through the Advisory Committee on Pesticides (ACP) which, as we have seen, consists of 'independent' experts and civil servants.[13] (For membership of this committee see appendix 10.) So far, there have been no fewer than nine referrals of 2,4,5-T to the ACP, and the overall conclusion of this committee has continued to be that the herbicide is safe so long as it is handled in accordance with instructions.

This view has been decisively rejected by the British trade union movement – a move which deserves particular attention here. It is a unique example of a firm political stance being taken in Britain to challenge the judgement of a supposedly independent and expert advisory committee, and indeed to assert a total lack of confidence in the procedures for the regulation of toxic chemicals, such as pesticides.

A key stage in the trade union campaign came in November 1979, when the National Union of Agricultural and Allied Workers (NUAAW) instructed its members at the Forestry Commission, and strongly advised its farmworker members, not to use 2,4,5-T. In March 1980, the NUAAW presented the then Minister of Agriculture, Peter Walker, with a dossier on the herbicide entitled *Not One Minute Longer*.[14] This gave details of a whole series of human cases where exposure to 2,4,5-T had been followed by toxic effects such as miscarriages, birth defects and sterility. The dossier also discounted the ACP's insistence that 2,4,5-T is safe so long as it is properly used:

It is the NUAAW's conviction, distilled from the experience of thousands of members working in forests and on farms that the conditions envisaged by members of the ACP (presumably used to the controlled conditions of the laboratory) are impossible to reproduce in the field.

This single fact must be sufficient to demolish the supposition that the herbicide is safe to use.[15]

In defiance of the ACP's claim for the safety of 2,4,5-T, by January 1980 a total of ten trade unions had united within the TUC to fight for a ban. In February, this policy was approved by the TUC General Council as a whole. A number of local authorities agreed to cease spraying of the herbicide (more than 70 are now in compliance with this), and these were joined by other major users such as British Rail, the Water Authorities Board, the National Coal Board and the Central Electricity Generating Board.

2,4,5-T itself is no longer manufactured in Britain, but is imported mainly from Germany. The ACP claimed in its March 1979 review that a mere 3 tonnes were used annually in the UK. However, according to customs and excise figures obtained by Labour MP Roger Thomas, a total of 116 tonnes were imported in 1979, and the British Agrochemicals Association (BAA) later admitted that about 58 tonnes of the active ingredient were sprayed in that year. More recent reports from the BAA suggest that total imports for 1979 may well have been as high as 164 tonnes. As a result of these disclosures, Thomas has accused the agrochemicals industry of 'gross deceit', and has urged the setting up of an inquiry with a view to establishing the full extent of the use of 2,4,5-T.[16] In May 1980, apparently in an attempt to alleviate anxiety over the chemical's continued use, the government suddenly announced a reduction in the permitted level of TCDD in 2,4,5-T from a maximum of 0.1 to 0.01 ppm. However, this has done nothing to diminish demands for a total ban.

In June 1980, and in response to mounting criticism of the APC's handling of the 2,4,5-T issue, a meeting was held between representatives of those unions most involved and the scientific sub-committee of the ACP. This confrontation lasted three-and-a-half hours, and the subcommittee members were made vividly aware of the total opposition of the trade unionists both to the assertion that certain levels of exposure to 2,4,5-T are 'acceptable' and also to the non-representative nature of the committee itself. The trade union representatives argued that the level of proof required in such cases should not be that of 'beyond all reasonable doubt' but rather of what is 'most likely on the balance of probabilities'.

At a subsequent meeting with the minister and several members of the ACP, some trade union representatives pointed out that the 2,4,5-T issue was now losing its significance, since many of the major users had banned it themselves. However, although 2,4,5-T use has greatly diminished, there remain unprotected groups who may still be exposed, including farmworkers, non-unionised workers, amateur gardeners, and certain local authority employees. Moreover, trade unionists emphasised at this second meeting that 2,4,5-T was only the first of a number of pesticides that would be the subject of major campaigns if the method of controlling pesticides was not drastically amended to include outside representation. The trade union representatives argued that a vital feature of this new regulatory structure should be the removal of responsibility for control from the purview of MAFF, whose concern with improving crop production seemed to take precedence over efforts to ensure the safety of farmworkers and the general public.

As further support for the arguments put by trade union representatives in these two meetings, TUC delegates at their annual congress, in September 1980, unanimously passed the following resolution:[17]

The campaign to ban the use of the weedkiller 2,4,5-T in Britain has exposed the system of control of pesticides to be a shambles. Congress calls for the Health and Safety Commission to take over responsibility for decisions on the safety and control of pesticides – a move which would involve the winding up of the Ministry of Agriculture's Pesticides Advisory Committee. Congress also reaffirms the TUC demand for the Government to ban the use of 2,4,5-T.

In December 1980, the most recent report of the ACP on 2,4,5-T was published.[18] As expected, this report was somewhat more comprehensive than its predecessors, but still indicated no major change in the official view of the herbicide's safety. The report suggested that no conclusive evidence of the health hazards of 2,4,5-T exists, and minimised the significance of human case studies such as those produced by the NUAAW. The trade union reply to this is to point to the wide range of known toxic effects on animals and the known or suspected effects on human beings.* In this situation, they claim, it is more than reasonable, 'on the balance of probabilities', to call for an immediate emergency ban whilst systematic studies of the long- and short-term hazards could be conducted – if indeed any further evidence is required.

On 17 December 1980 (immediately after publication of the ACP report), the TUC General Council voted unanimously to stop 2,4,5-T coming into the country through Britain's docks, and to trace foreign manufacturing sites so as to encourage overseas trade unions to cease production. This decision represents a new commitment by the British trade union movement to the protection of the workforce and the environment. The TUC is not only telling the government to ban a chemical, but is also expressing a complete lack of confidence in the existing expert advisory committees and demanding new policies – not just on one single issue, but for a whole category of substances.

The 2,4,5-T controversy illustrates a number of general features of the British control of toxic substances. In particular, it shows the huge gap between the approaches taken by the official advisory committee – which seems content to await indefinitely the arrival of *conclusive* proof of toxicity – and by the trade union movement – which has demanded a more cautious approach, consistent with established principles of public health. The insistence by trade unions that they must participate in decisions of this sort is also important, since it suggests a growing lack of faith in the now traditional British policy of 'leaving it to the experts'. As we have seen, 2,4,5-T has been the subject of unprecedented action by the whole trade union movement in seeking to protect the interests of its members and the general public. The militant action conducted in

---

* Perhaps the most graphic reply came from NUAAW general secretary, Jack Boddy, who declared: 'This review is a monstrous whitewash. But whitewash gets thinner at the ninth time of using and no one will be fooled this time. Whitewash is no antidote to poison.'

regard to 2,4,5-T has been based on a united approach by a number of trade unions and, as such, it could well provide a model for future campaigns on issues of health and safety.

In 1982, a book was published which recounts in some detail the 'story' of 2,4,5-T and draws on trade union experience of the issue to propose a 'charter for the safer use of pesticides'.[19] Apart from demanding an immediate ban in Britain on the use of 2,4,5-T, the charter calls for:

- The abolition of the ACP – responsibility for the clearance of pesticides to be transferred to the HSE.
- The replacement of the various *voluntary* schemes for the control of pesticide usage by a *statutory* scheme.
- Stricter standards of pesticide control and the better enforcement of regulations (e.g. by the appointment of worker safety representatives in agriculture).
- No new pesticides to be licensed without proof of efficacy.
- Increased research into techniques of pest management that reduce the use of chemical pesticides.
- The establishment of a British version of the American Environment Protection Agency, independent of government and industry.

This charter provides a good starting-point for any discussion and action on the future control of *all* hazardous pesticides.

7. How industry resists regulation*

This chapter reviews the ways in which industry resists regulation, drawing examples from previous case studies. There are many strategies used by British industry to delay the drawing up of regulations or to restrict their effectiveness when implemented, and we will describe some of them here. These tactics are often similar to those used by firms in the USA – but inevitably there are also differences, reflecting the differences in the regulatory systems of the two countries. Perhaps the most significant of these are that the British system is much more closed and secretive than its American counterpart and that there is a relative lack of well-informed opposition from trade unions and environmental groups backed by an independent scientific community.

Playing down the risk

Through this strategy, industry aims to alleviate public concern and to argue that the cost of 'unreasonable' control of a carcinogen would be prohibitive. A standard argument is to blame present cases of cancer on high *past* levels of exposure to occupational carcinogens – the implication being that workers are now much safer since exposure has been reduced. In this way, debate about the real dangers of current levels of exposure is avoided. Another tactic is to focus attention on 'proven' human carcinogens only. Epidemiological proof of human carcinogenicity is difficult to obtain, especially in occupational groups which are often small, with high turnover rates, and where exposure data have not been

* This chapter is based on and incorporates material from chapter 10 of S. Epstein, *The Politics of Cancer*, Anchor Press, New York (1979).

collected or are not made available. In the case of VC, for instance, attention was centred on the rare example of angiosarcoma of the liver – which could not be denied – while evidence of its causing other more common cancers, particularly of the lung, brain and digestive tract, was ignored or discounted.

Numbers games

Another technique is the comparison of risks on some numerical scale in order to demonstrate that it is unreasonable to worry about the risk of an occupational cancer when we happily accept the day-to-day risks of smoking, crossing the road, flying, and such like. One development of this technique has been to propose an 'index of risk' for those activities which we 'choose' to undertake. Widely differing pursuits such as travelling by car, staying at home or working in different industries can then be compared – often in terms of their Fatal Accident Frequency Rate (FAFR). FAFR is defined as the number of fatal accidents in a group of 1,000 people in a working lifetime (taken as 100 million hours). How then, industrialists argue, can one mount a rational case for improvements in the safety of British industry when its overall FAFR is 4, compared with 57 for travelling by car or 5 for travelling by train?[1]

A number of points can be made in reply to such arguments. First of all, one can criticise the statistical data on which such comparisons are made. Deaths on the roads can be counted all too easily, a clear cause–effect relationship can be identified and historical experience provides a solid basis for the prediction of annual death rates in the future. As we have seen, occupational cancer deaths are far less easy to count, cause-effect relationships are difficult to pinpoint and wide disagreement exists over the future incidence of morbidity and mortality. Accordingly, numerical comparisons are likely to be extremely misleading.

Secondly, one can suggest that the existence of greater evils in no way diminishes the need to reduce the number of avoidable deaths from cancer. A related point is made by Judith Cook and Chris Kaufman in their argument for a ban on 2,4,5-T: 'We are told that there are far more dangerous farm chemicals around and that motor cars cause more havoc. If that is so, then let us see campaigns on these issues too.'[2]

The third point is that the 'numbers game' seems to assume that it is possible to compare risks on a numerical scale when they may have been undertaken in different social circumstances and for quite different reasons. Some risks may legitimately be labelled 'voluntary' (e.g. rock climbing), but others, such as working in a hazardous industry, can hardly be termed a 'free choice' when there may be few alternative sources of employment. Chronic and acute effects may also be evaluated differently, and certain effects – such as cancer – cause particular worry. Different risks are not therefore strictly comparable, and whilst narrow statistical comparisons may occasionally serve to highlight areas for concern, they are, in general, misleading. In particular, they neglect the real situations involved and the distribution of benefits and costs. It is also important to stress that blanket terms such as FAFR tend to disguise three possible areas of inequality regarding risk – *social* inequality (the fact that certain classes are disproportionally affected); *geographical* inequality (risks are unevenly distributed in national and international terms); and *temporal* inequality (the possibility that future generations will suffer the consequences of hazards over which they have no control whatsoever).

One other, associated, industrial tactic is to insist on degrees of scientific precision in carcinogenicity tests and epidemiological studies that cannot be met. As we have seen, such a strategy usually entails insistence on awaiting results of prospective long-term human studies before the introduction of stricter regulation is considered. In the USA, where regulation is determined by a standard developed in open hearing, these arguments are used as a routine delaying tactic. In Britain, they are often used against 'unnecessarily strict' hygiene standards being introduced in a code of practice. In the case of VC, for instance, the debate which British industry wanted to have was:

Whether any residual risk remained once exposure had been reduced to the 1–10 ppm range, whether any significant quantifiable reduction of risk occurred within this range by reducing vinyl chloride levels from below 10 ppm to 1 ppm and whether the use of respirators to achieve the lower of these introduced a greater, albeit small, risk of death from fire or explosion.[3]

Such a debate would inevitably be protracted by experts attempting to discern any long-term trends in the statistics. Indeed, it could well be impossible to resolve, and, in the meantime, the industry would continue to work to the less strict standard.

Technological arrogance

Industry believes that most carcinogenic risk can be successfully controlled by technology and managerial competence – prohibition is an outmoded approach, according to the CIA. However, ICI thought this to be the case almost 30 years ago, when they constructed a new 'safe' plant for the manufacture of alpha-naphthylamine. It was closed after discovery of the first cases of bladder cancer which the plant had been designed to avoid. Each epoch is characterised by industry's renewed 'technological arrogance' which can only be proved inadequate after a further 20–30 years' experience. The unions argue that risk cannot be reduced to negligible levels in practice, because of human fallibility and the pursuit of production and profit, but that some risks may be 'acceptable' if the benefits to the risk-takers and society are great enough. Where they are not, then prohibition will be necessary.

'Throw them a hostage'

When the evidence about the carcinogenicity of several substances is strong, but particularly overwhelming in the case of one substance, then industry may sacrifice that substance by banning it as a carcinogen, thereby shifting attention from the other, more economically viable, substances. The most obvious example is asbestos. All types were considered dangerous up until about 1955–60, when mesothelioma came to be associated more with blue than white or brown asbestos. Although all asbestos types had previously been associated with asbestosis and lung cancer, they soon came to be regarded as 'safe', once the idea that 'blue is dangerous' took hold of popular consciousness, via industry propaganda. Another example comes from the history of the aromatic amines, where the chemical companies seized upon beta-naphthylamine as the culprit, in order to protect other substances under suspicion, such as benzidine.

This tactic can also be used when a process is under suspicion – the 'old' process is regarded as the problem, and the new process excused from all blame. This tactic was used by town gas manufacturers who, on receiving Richard Doll's first evidence of cancer amongst their workers, decided that it was the old, horizontal retort houses that had caused the problem, and not the more recent vertical retort houses. It took a further 20 years to establish that both types contributed to excess cancer. By that time, the industry was finished, having been replaced by North Sea Gas.

Influencing policy

In the USA, lobbyists for industry, particularly trade associations such as the Chemical Manufacturers' Association, combine with sympathetic congressmen to form a very efficient lobbying organisation which presents evidence at hearings in an attempt to affect regulatory proceedings in favour of industry. In Britain, there is less opportunity for such adversarial campaigns, but industrial trade associations such as the Chemical Industries Association (CIA) do play a significant part in policy-making. The CIA co-ordinates the chemical industries' representation in any discussions. A small but powerful secretariat, its strength lies in the relationship it has built up with government through its technical and medical work produced by experts available from member companies. On sensitive issues such as suspected or proven carcinogens, the CIA also handles the media representation for the industry and has built up considerable skill in this area. The scale of its activities in the VC case, for example, was considerable. It was also instrumental in blocking the Health and Safety Commission's (HSC) scheme for pre-market notification of new chemicals in favour of the considerably weaker scheme proposed by the EEC for all member states (see chapter 3).

Exhausting the system

The nature of the regulatory system in the USA is such that it is possible for industry to delay the introduction of regulations by taking legal action, the costs of such action usually being more than offset by the continued profit from sales. As a result, industry tries to enforce a case-by-case approach and has resisted attempts by OSHA to introduce a 'generic' approach for all occupational carcinogens.

In Britain, both government and industry have, until recently, agreed that each case should be treated separately and there has been no real move towards developing a standard policy for all carcinogens. Moreover, there is no legal redress should a standard be set which a trade union, for instance, rejects. In the particular case of exposure to carcinogens, as with other occupational hazards, once the problem is recognised, a standard is supposed to be developed by government, industry and unions reaching a consensus on scientific data. Should such a new standard be agreed, then presumably it will be heeded. The difficulty is that management and unions often fail to agree, and, while the argument goes on, the old standard continues to be used. Although the first VC standard of 10 ppm over an eight-hour working day was quickly agreed to, the system has not run so smoothly since and it has proved much harder to achieve consensus on the major advisory committees of the HSC, as trade union representatives have become more confident in taking a strong line.

The most interesting example of disagreements within this system is the recent split between the HSC and its enforcing body, the HSE, over a policy for occupational carcinogens (see chapter 3). But whatever the outcome of the present disagreements, it is likely that industry will be able to exhaust any new system devised, and the position which the CIA has taken over carcinogen control is very interesting in this respect.[4] They concede, reluctantly, that separate carcinogen regulations *will* be required, both because proposals from the EEC have already been taken up in other EEC member states and because trade unions seem to be insisting on such an approach. Having said this, however, they then go on to propose a three-stage control process which keeps the most important decisions firmly under their control. The first two stages are assessment of the degree of carcinogenic hazard, based on the study of animal experiments and medical data, and assessment of the degree of risk based on methods and scale of manufacture or use of the carcinogen. Both of these stages would be the job of small groups of experts (in so-called 'Hazard and Risk Assessment Committees'). Given the uncertainty of so much of the relevant information, these committees could take a very long time to come to a conclusion. Only when they did so would the individual case then be passed on to the tripartite decision-making structure for a judgement to be made, based on the expert advice emerging from the first two stages.

It is clear that such a system would have immense potential for spinning out the procedure for drawing up regulations to control each individual suspected carcinogen. Such proposals would also ensure that much of the discussion on the balancing of incomplete data on carcinogenic risk against highly contentious data on the 'costs' to industry of strict controls, took place within small groups of experts which excluded lay people, such as the workers or consumers exposed to the carcinogen.

Controlling the information

Another problem with the present system which would be intensified by the CIA's proposals is that it is likely that many of the experts called upon to serve on the suggested Hazard and Risk Assessment Committees would themselves have close contacts with the industry they would be regulating. An allied point is that most of the information on which decisions are made is produced or controlled by industry. There is no effective body of trade-union-funded, or community-backed research in Britain. Coupled with traditional secrecy of government and of industries in competitive markets, this means that there is little encouragement to researchers to blow the whistle on research which they feel to be inadequate, misused, or even fraudulent. As a result, trade unionists and other activists often have to rely on American data which the industries concerned may then attack as irrelevant to

Britain. The case of VC provides a good example of this, since, as we have seen, it was the British Society for Social Responsibility in Science and the unions who passed on to the workers the information available to them from the USA.[5]

In Britain, it is very difficult to discover just what information is being used by industry to reach decisions relating to the health and safety of its products and processes. A recent example was the discovery by the Manchester Area Safety Committee (MASC)* that a senior toxicologist in ICI was apparently not aware of a 'Current Intelligence Bulletin' from NIOSH which gave details of animal carcinogenicity tests on a group of chemicals called chloroethanes, many of which ICI uses or makes in large quantities.[6] The most common of these is 1,1,1-trichlorethane, the main constituent of ICI's solvent 'Genklene'. Although this chemical had not yet been proven carcinogenic in the tests, caution was urged by NIOSH until further testing could be completed. Only after circulating this information did MASC discover ICI's apparent ignorance of the NIOSH Bulletin. ICI, however, produced a counter-document seemingly designed to play down the risk, using the results of tests done by an American competitor, Dow Chemical.

The response of the CIA to the 1980 ASTMS policy document[7] on cancer was also revealing. Two CIA documents were produced. One was a review of the ASTMS document which basically attacked the scientific evidence presented in the pamphlet and tried to portray it as too extreme to be countenanced by any experts except those with a political axe to grind.[8] The same idea was reinforced by the second CIA document entitled *Cancer in Modern Mortality*,[9] in which the claim that occupation is responsible for much less than 5 per cent of cancers was presented as hard fact rather than a controversial estimate.

The CIA's anxiety about increasing union concern over occupational cancer was also demonstrated by its reaction to the GMWU's Preliminary Cancer Prevention Programme in 1979. In

---

* MASC was one of the many local health and safety organisations formed by trade union branches and shop stewards' committees in the late 1970s. For a current list of these groups see appendix 7.

this programme, the union drew attention to what appeared to be the rising trend of cancer in the UK, and to the substantial evidence of carcinogenicity in over 100 chemical substances collected by the International Agency for Research on Cancer (IARC). It then circulated the IARC list to the top 20 chemical companies and to the CIA, asking them for their policies towards animal and human carcinogens, their control methods, and their provision of information to workers and customers. The CIA reacted by advising member companies not to respond to the alarmist and 'ill-informed' GMWU letter, saying that it was being dealt with at national level.

The GMWU then sent the policy and similar questions to its shop stewards and safety representatives in the chemical industry. The CIA asked its member companies 'to refrain from responding to the union's questions', because it would give rise to 'further confusion and probably to unnecessary alarm'. The 'joint investigations' promised at national level did not take place. The CIA was again successful and very few safety representatives received answers to their questions. Meanwhile, the CIA had set about producing a policy on occupational carcinogens which it published in December 1981, some three years after the unions had asked for it.[10] In their reply, ASTMS and GMWU rejected the CIA's approach, which they see as being designed more to preserve industry's freedom to use carcinogenic substances than to prevent occupational cancer. The unions argue that a generic approach is essential (utilising the existing evaluations of the IARC), that separate regulatory treatment of carcinogenic substances is necessary and that the whole process of hazard and risk evaluation should involve workers' representatives.[11]

By November 1982, no real dialogue on occupational cancer had yet occurred between the main unions involved in the debate – GMWU and ASTMS – and the CIA. This failure was due in part to CIA's insistence that their expert doctors could talk to union doctors only, and not to medically unqualified union health and safety officers.

Propagandising the public

In the USA, much time and money is spent by industry on trying to convince the public that particular carcinogens are not really dangerous. Indeed, a campaign by an industry organisation called the Calorie Control Council to defend saccharin was so successful that the resulting outcry led to a moratorium on the regulation to ban it. The situation in Britain has traditionally been somewhat different. Largely because of the closed nature of the regulatory system, there are no obvious examples of this kind. However, the climate is now changing and some industries are worried about the public image of their products. For instance, the outcry produced by the revelation of the dangers of asbestos in the mid-1970s led the Asbestos Information Committee (an industry-funded body) to run an advertising campaign estimated to have cost £500,000.[12] This consisted of a series of full-page advertisements in national newspapers and a poster campaign telling the public how safe, useful, clean, and cheap asbestos is, if used properly. Little was said about the hazards of asbestos, and the principal arguments used to gain public support centred on the supposed 'miracle' properties of asbestos in fire and accident prevention.

Apart from specific campaigns of this kind, an increasing amount of money is being spent by those industries which feel most threatened to get their version of reality across to the public. Indeed, the CIA describes 'external relations and public education'[13] as the second main priority of its Chemical Industry Safety and Health Council. Television and newspapers often carry advertising campaigns from large chemical or drug companies which are not concerned at all with the possible hazards of products. Instead, such publicity focuses on the dynamism of the companies, the importance of their products for the quality of life, or the care which they supposedly show for the environment.

Blaming the victim

An additional way of avoiding responsibility for the real problems of occupationally induced cancer is to suggest that anyone who does contract an industrial disease must be at fault themselves, since industry has done all it can to ensure the health and safety of its workers. Two versions of this argument are commonly used: the first refers to the genetic make-up of the worker; the second blames the worker's personal habits. Interestingly, a recent article in the *British Medical Journal* reported that both genetic and life-style factors are now being sought to explain bladder cancer – one of the earliest forms of cancer to be related to occupation.[14]

The idea that some workers are 'hypersusceptible' to cancer and should not be allowed to work where they might be exposed to carcinogenic substances may have some superficial plausibility and has obvious attractions for some industries. However, in reality, it is a very dangerous argument (see appendix 3). There is no evidence that any work-related cancer can be explained away in this fashion – indeed, it would be very difficult to gather enough data to prove, or to disprove, such a notion. More importantly, the effect of the acceptance of this highly speculative approach would be to shift attention away from the question 'Which chemicals cause cancer?' to 'Which people get cancer?', thereby legitimating the continued exposure of allegedly more resistant workers to high levels of carcinogens.

The other 'blaming the victim' argument emphasises 'life-style' rather than occupational exposure to chemicals. The 'careless worker' has figured frequently in explanations of high accident rates and workers who contract illnesses are often blamed for not taking the proper precautions. Furthermore, smoking is held by some to be exclusively responsible for lung cancer. Everyone, except the tobacco industry, recognises that smoking is the main factor in many lung cancers, but, in the case of asbestos at least, it is clear that workers who smoke are *more* likely to develop cancer when they are also exposed to dust. Moreover, a substantial number of non-smokers also develop lung cancer, while mesothelioma, the other main asbestos-related cancer, has little if any association with smoking. Many industrial dusts, chemicals and processes are now proven or suspected causes of lung cancer – irrespective of whether the victims smoke or not (see appendix 3).

The flight of the multinationals

In the USA, when regulation was carried out at the state level, dangerous and polluting industrial processes were moved to the southern states where control was more lax. With the introduction of federal legislation, new standards have made production more costly so that 'runaway' factories – asbestos plants, for instance – have been set up over the Mexican border, in the Far East, or in Eastern Europe. Furthermore, some products have been banned on health grounds in the USA, yet continue to be exported – especially to the third world. Examples of such 'corporate dumping' include pesticides, drugs and various contraceptive devices.[15]

In this country, the picture is more complicated. On the one hand, there are examples of substances and processes being imported into Britain to take advantage of standards which are relatively laxer than their American counterparts. Production of the pesticide dibromochloropropane (DBCP), for instance, is banned in the USA since the chemical is known to cause sterility as well as being carcinogenic. In this country, it has also failed to get clearance from the government pesticide scheme, but the British scheme is only voluntary and production of DBCP still continues at several places in this country for export, mainly to the third world.[16]

There are also examples where production has been removed from Britain as British standards have toughened or as attitudes have changed. The most notorious example of this is probably the production and use of blue asbestos products which are now banned in this country, but are still common in third world countries. Even in the 1930s when the hazards of asbestos were first brought to light, one of the big British companies set up production in northern France to take advantage of a more compliant workforce.[17]

A recent example, publicised by *New Scientist*,[18] is the provision of the pesticide aldrin by British American Tobacco (BAT) to Kenyan farmers. Tobacco is now the main cash crop in Kenya and vast quantities of insecticide are needed to protect it. *New Scientist* pointed out that the leaflet of precautions issued with the pesticide was useless, given the rural isolation of many of the farms, and that contamination of water supplies by pesticides is a real problem. Following the *New Scientist* report, BAT announced that they were withdrawing aldrin supplies from the farmers, but the alternative they were using – a chemical called orthene – also requires more stringent precautions than could realistically be expected. It is particularly ironic that the company concerned should be BAT – the world's largest tobacco company. In 1982, it was calculated that BAT's turnover during the year would top £4,000 million, much of it from trade in the developing countries, where its sales efforts are not hampered by advertising restrictions.[19] In Kenya, for instance, BAT has a monopoly over tobacco production. It does not run farms itself but contracts out to 8,500 farmers, mainly with small farms in remote areas, who grow the tobacco in return for credit, seeds, supplies and advice from the company. Not only does the tobacco cash crop take up valuable land and labour which could be used for growing food, but it also fails to generate much export capital since BAT's policy is to produce for domestic markets only. Of course, BAT is not the only company implicated in such practices. Other companies sell pesticides containing aldrin, and use advertising which would not be acceptable in Britain. Britain is currently one of the largest exporters of pesticides to the third world, supplying over 12 per cent of the world market.

Playing up the costs of regulation

This strategy is one which is likely to become increasingly important in Britain. Basically, the arguments used are first that it would cost too much to reduce the risk from a particular substance to a given level and second that stringent requirements for pre-market testing will act as an obstacle to innovation. Both practices are said to render the industry less competitive, thereby putting jobs at risk. In the USA, where product testing is already legally required and where standards set for carcinogens have generally been stricter than in Britain, industry has been putting forward this argument for some time. In Britain, the situation is still confused (as we have seen in chapter 3), but whatever the outcome of present arguments, we do know that some system of testing and control will have to come in future legislation; already, industry has started to raise arguments similar to those used in the USA about the disincentive effects of strict pre-market testing and product-liability laws.[20]

It is interesting, therefore, that a number of American studies have recently been published which show that stricter regulation can actually have a *beneficial* effect on industrial innovation.[21] As Ashford and Heaton put it:

> The regulations having to do with safety and environment seemed to be a *positive stimulus* to commercial innovation in a significant number of cases, especially in mature and concentrated industries i.e. automobiles and chemicals.[22]

In particular, pollution controls force companies to think about recycling effluents. British Distilleries, for example, decided to recycle their still-bottom wastes, and received a 100 per cent return on their resulting investment in animal foods in one year.[23]

In 1981, the National Economic Development Organisation (NEDO) attempted to identify the costs and benefits of health, safety and environmental controls to British chemical companies, but the questionnaires to companies showed that they had little idea of costs or benefits. NEDO concluded that, 'in general, companies believe that the level of costs incurred at present is appropriate to the benefits obtained.'[24] In evidence submitted to the NEDO study, the GMWU suggested that there were at least eleven benefits to industry from health, safety and environmental controls, ranging from improved throughput efficiencies and reduced wastage of raw materials, to improved productivity and marketing potential.

In this chapter we have demonstrated the many strategies employed by industry to resist regulation and have shown how this can often be detrimental to the health of workers and consumers. In the final chapter we discuss strategies for fighting back.

8. How to fight back: the politics of prevention*

Cancer is not just a 'natural' and unavoidable problem. It is a disease which often has social and economic causes. Moreover, it affects different groups in the population disproportionately, so that those with the least power and the fewest resources are also most likely to become its victims. It follows, therefore, that the fight against cancer and the prevention of the disease will involve individuals, families and groups consciously changing some of the ways in which they live their lives. But, more importantly, it will involve many different forms of *collective* action. Thus the cancer problem cannot be relegated to the 'experts' or to the economically self-interested, but has to be shifted to the wider political arena where it more properly belongs.

Individual strategies to reduce your exposure to carcinogens

We begin with some basic suggestions about ways in which individuals can try to minimise their exposure to avoidable carcinogens. We realise, however, that this may be very difficult to achieve. Often, people are not even aware of the risks they are running, since information on the carcinogenicity of a given substance may either not be known or be unavailable to the public. Moreover, even when people *are* aware of a risk, they may be unable to do anything about it, since, for most people, freedom of action is limited by the paramount need to make a living. Thus, it may be extremely difficult for someone to change their job or to move house however dangerous they may suspect their present

---

* This chapter is based on and incorporates material from chapter 11 of
  S. Epstein, *The Politics of Cancer*, Anchor Press, New York (1979).

environment to be. Similarly, the inability to give up smoking will be strongly influenced by the stresses of daily life and the availability of alternative sources of satisfaction and enjoyment. However, despite these limitations, it is important to list the main ways in which people can try to avoid exposure to carcinogens and thereby reduce their chances of contracting cancer. Not only are such strategies likely to keep them healthier, but they are also one form of direct action against those corporate interests which place profit before health.

The work you do

Your place of work can greatly affect your chances of getting cancer. Workers in petrochemical, asbestos, steel-smelting and some mining industries are particularly high-risk groups (see appendix 1). While the risks are greatest in these basic-manu-facturing industries, they also extend to those industries which fabricate or use these basic products to make other goods. For people already employed in high-risk industries, it is important to be actively involved in your union and to ensure that it fights to reduce carcinogenic and other toxic hazards in your own work-place as well as campaigning for a tightening of the regulations at the national level. Some unions (in particular, ASTMS, GMWU and NGA) are now beginning to advise their members to negotiate 'no carcinogens' agreements with their employers (there is an example of such an agreement in appendix 5). You should try to find out the position of your own union and, if necessary, press for more priority to be given to such issues. As a first step, insist that your employer identifies to you any of the established animal or human carcinogens in your workplace; ensure that your employer's processes are such that there is minimal or no risk of exposure to the workforce (see appendix 1; a very useful book is *Cancer and Work*, City University Statistical Laboratory and GMWU, 1983). Let your GP know (and get it on your medical record) if you are or have been exposed to any of these carcinogens.

Of course, any policy to restrict the use of carcinogenic materials might produce problems for workers in other industries. They may see demand for their products drop, thus threatening their liveli-hoods (for example, asbestos workers would clearly suffer from an immediate ban or even a rapid phase-out of asbestos products). This is why cancer is as much an economic and political issue as it is a medical and scientific one. Pressure to remove dangerous chemicals from workplaces means putting health higher up the scale of trade union priorities, and campaigns need to be fought to replace dangerous processes and products with less hazardous ones which could still keep people in work. In short, the campaign for alternative products and processes, which is already under way in industries threatened by rationalisation and closure, needs to be linked with the struggle against ill-health and, particularly, against cancer. This is especially vital for workers in the tobacco industry.

Where you live

More and more people are now having to live near chemical plants, refineries, or hazardous-waste disposal sites, as well as heavily used main roads or motorways. Not only can such environments be aesthetically unpleasant, but they may also pose serious health risks. It is important to try and find out about any possible risk from the emission of industrial carcinogens into your local community and either join – or, if necessary, initiate – a local group to fight pollution of this kind. Important examples of such campaigns have occurred recently in Ireland, where many inhabitants of the area around Cork fought against the siting of an asbestos plant in their community by the American firm Raybestos Manhattan. Several other local communities have now formed action groups to fight against the dumping of toxic wastes in their locality, and one of the most successful of these campaigns has been run by the inhabitants of Finglas – a working-class suburb of Dublin.[1]

It is important to emphasise that local campaigns may not necessarily be directed against industrial firms. Some toxic-waste dumps have been officially supported by local councils, and groups in various parts of the country have also been involved in struggles to force their local authority to deal with the dangerous asbestos used in some garages, council houses, hospitals, schools and other public buildings. In April 1976, it was found that more than 200 people on the modern Samuel Pepys council estate in south London had been exposed to deadly blue asbestos. It was only after continuing demands from the tenants that the council undertook proper investigations and carried out repairs to seal off the ceilings.[2]

Your smoking habits

It is perfectly true that the most effective *single* action you can take to reduce your chances of getting cancer is either not to take up smoking or – if you have already done so – to give it up as quickly as possible. There is no real alternative to quitting – switching to low-tar brands, or to cigars or a pipe, is *not* an effective method of avoiding cancer. However, quitting smoking should not be regarded simply as an individual's own responsibility, but needs to be part of a broader campaign. It is important, therefore, to argue against smoking in meetings and other gatherings – trade union branch meetings, for example – and to take a firm stand on the right of non-smokers to clean air in public places – including workplaces. The evidence about 'passive smoking' works well and overcomes arguments like: 'Why are you denying me my rights when it doesn't affect you?' At the same time, it is also important to press your union or employer to provide educational and support services for those smokers who wish to give up.

Medical treatment

X-rays are potentially carcinogenic, so you should try to avoid any that are not absolutely necessary. Obviously, most people find it very difficult to question their doctor's decisions and the number of unnecessary medical X-rays performed in Britain is probably far less than in the USA. However, it is always important to be clear about the nature of any medical procedure you may be required to undergo and – if necessary – to try and make some assessment of its potential value compared with any possible risks. Frequent chest X-rays, for example, are often of very limited value in identifying industrial diseases, and can be a source of false reassurance. Routine dental X-rays have also become a matter for concern in Britain. In many instances their diagnostic value is doubtful and they are often performed with old machines in less than ideal conditions.

Similarly, it is extremely important to try and find out as much as you can about any drug that is prescribed for you. There are certainly circumstances under which a carcinogenic drug may be worth the risk – for the treatment of a life-threatening condition, for example. However, you should consider whether or not it is worth taking such a drug for less serious conditions, particularly over a long period. You should always ask your doctor about the side-effects of any drug you may be given. If you are not *entirely* satisfied with his/her advice, you should seek further information from one of the consumer guides to medicines.[3]

A woman who is experiencing the menopause may well have distressing symptoms and the health workers with whom she comes into contact often have little sympathy with her problems. However, if you do find yourself in this situation, you should think very carefully before taking oestrogens; if you do, then stick to a low dose for as short a period as possible. If you are taking the contraceptive pill, you should consider the possibility of switching to another form of birth control, particularly if you smoke and are over 35, have been on the pill for a lengthy period of time or envisage using it on a long-term basis in the future. If your GP is not helpful in deciding on an alternative you should try your local family planning clinic, well women clinic or women's health group.[4]

The food you eat
For your general health, you should try to eat a diet which is low in animal fats and high in fibre. That is to say, you should avoid eating too many dairy products and high-fat meats and replace them with an adequate amount of fruit, vegetables and grains. In particular, avoid eating highly processed 'junk' foods, most of which are rich in chemical additives and low in nutritional value.

Your choice of consumer products
Try to avoid consumer products that may contain carcinogens – some of which we have already discussed in the case studies. This is often difficult because of inadequate labelling. You should be especially careful of pesticide formulations, a number of which are based on known carcinogens such as chlordane and heptachlor. It

has recently come to light that many of the herbicides in everyday domestic use contain 2,4,5-T, which is invariably contaminated with dioxin.[5]

It is also advisable not to use cleaning or degreasing agents and solvents containing carbon tetrachloride, trichloroethylene, perchloroethylene or benzene – all of which are toxic and either known or suspected carcinogens. Instead, use alternatives based on detergents. Be especially careful to avoid all do-it-yourself products containing asbestos.

So far, then, we have listed some of the ways in which we can all attempt to reduce our exposure to carcinogens. However, these individual solutions can only be of limited value. We therefore continue with some suggestions about the form that a more collective campaign for cancer prevention might take.

Political strategies to reduce exposure to carcinogens

Cancer is a problem that affects everyone. We all know at least one person who suffers or has died from cancer, and we all fear cancer for ourselves. It is important, therefore, to see the prevention of cancer as an issue that potentially could unite a wide range of individuals and groups with otherwise diverse interests. Trade unionists concerned with health and safety issues, anti-nuclear groups, national and local environmental groups, women's health groups, sections of scientific and medical communities, various consumer organisations and some parliamentary reform groups, such as the Freedom of Information Group, are all engaged in one way or another in the fight against cancer. But the efforts of these groups need to be more effectively integrated. Moreover, any campaign needs to involve the many thousands of people who might not see themselves as 'political' in the normal sense of the term, but who are only too aware of the devastation cancer causes – old-age pensioners or certain religious organisations, for example.

What would the goals of such a campaign be? Clearly, its major aim would be to eliminate, or at least reduce to a minimum, those cancers that are preventable. And, as we have seen, a large proportion of all cancers probably fit into this category. The first priority must therefore be the creation of an effective system for the control of all chemicals, both old and new, in the workplace and outside it.

The identification and regulation of carcinogens

An effective system can only be achieved if there is a rethinking of the basic principles upon which the regulation of carcinogens is based. This would involve some agreement on a set of criteria – and not only scientific criteria – for judging whether or not a given substance is to be regulated as a human risk. In part, this would mean deciding on the relative weights to be attached to epidemiological, long-term animal and short-term carcinogenicity test results. It would also mean that industry should be charged for the costs of testing its chemicals in independent laboratories. But, above all, any approach that was to be effective would need to be based not on the lengthy wait for human victims by epidemiology, but on the scientifically-informed position that *all* substances proven carcinogenic in animals pose a risk to humans. Of course, such a system might possibly deny clearance to the rare substances that were eventually shown not to cause cancer in humans – but such errors of caution would normally be justified by the lives that could be saved. Additionally, some consideration of the social usefulness of a product would also need to be involved at this stage of the regulatory process, with a view to restricting or banning dangerous and non-useful products, and substituting safer alternatives for dangerous but useful products. Obviously, the availability of safer substitutes depends at present on industry having developed alternative materials and this demonstrates the problems inherent in a situation where the state applies regulatory controls only on the *use* of existing materials without controlling the direction of industrial development. Further discussion is needed of the potential for state or popular action to make avoidance of hazards an essential requirement of research and development.

The next stage of an effective prevention policy would involve the use of these test results to draw up a schedule of substances either known or suspected to be carcinogens. Such a schedule would need to consist not only of carcinogens likely to be used in the workplace, but also those likely to be found in consumer products or in the general environment. Above all, such lists and the data from which they were constructed would need to be easily available to the public as a first step in the identification of possible hazards.

There would also need to be an effective regulatory process that could be initiated automatically whenever a new substance was added to the schedule. Such a process would, of course, also be applied continuously to all substances already identified as carcinogens. An approach of this kind could be applied to both old and new chemicals, with a licensing procedure to prevent *new* carcinogens being brought into use. The difficulties of dealing with the thousands of chemicals already in use are obviously more daunting, but we can no longer afford to ignore them. Thus, while it would probably be impracticable to test them all in the immediate future a scheme is urgently needed to review all the toxicological information at present available on these substances – preferably through international co-operation – while a more effective monitoring system would enable possible hazards to be detected earlier. Additionally, a system of priorities should be established for the testing of those untested chemicals already in common use.

The setting up of mechanisms of this kind for identifying possible carcinogens and establishing control limits would then need to be followed up by the creation of an effective system of enforcement to ensure that no carcinogens were being used illegally or under hazardous conditions. But in discussing enforcement we need to say something more about the notion of 'banning' chemicals. If, as seems clear, there is no level of exposure below which cancers cannot be induced, then it is arguable that all known carcinogens should be banned. Not surprisingly, the Chemical Industries Association, representing corporate industrial opinion, is firmly against such a view – at least as far as occupational carcinogens are concerned. Indeed, they have recently stated that

prohibition or banning are essentially outmoded approaches, because effective control measures may be developed to contain the most toxic materials or processes, whether that toxicity is acute or chronic. Once the conditions of production or use have been laid down, it will be economic considerations that will largely determine whether the required control technology can be applied and whether the material or process will be retained in use.[6]

It is certainly true that a sudden ban on some carcinogens would come up against strong opposition, not only from profit-seeking industrialists but also from workers whose jobs are at stake if a particular carcinogen can no longer be manufactured or used. Thus, to ban or not to ban should not be decided as a once-and-for-all principle. When an industrial chemical is of obvious social value (either potentially or because it is already a major industrial material), and where control of this chemical is easy, then a straightforward banning may in fact be too rigid a policy. This will occur when the processes in which the chemical is made or used are readily containable and easy to monitor, when the industry has large numbers of well-trained safety officers kept on their toes by vigilant trade union safety representatives, and when the chemicals are made or used in a small number of modern establishments easily overseen by the Factory Inspectorate. It could be argued, though many would disagree, that this is now the case with vinyl chloride – so long as attempts are continually made to reduce concentrations of VC in workplace air.

However, there are many other chemicals to which these conditions do not apply because the products themselves may be marginal in their social value; standards of hygiene and safety in the industry may be low; unions may be fragmented and weak; the process may be technically difficult to contain; and/or the chemical may be so widespread in use that there are too many workplaces for the Factory Inspectorate to police. In such cases (and asbestos and 2,4,5-T are both good examples), the straightforward banning of a substance and its substitution with other products *does* make sense. This shows how discussions of control measures for carcinogens must take into account the structure of the industry, and the feasibility of actually enforcing the regulations. If the appropriate regulations *cannot* be enforced, then weakening them to suit industrial interests is not the answer. The chemical concerned must be banned.

So far, we have been concerned only with the banning of chemicals in use in the workplace. When we turn to the use of potentially carcinogenic chemicals in consumer products and in the wider environment, questions relating to potential risks and benefits often become even more complex and difficult to assess, and the lack of effective enforcement mechanisms may well make a ban the only reasonable strategy.

At present, certain areas of enforcement are relatively strong – in the case of food additives or drugs, for instance – but others, relating to the workplace and the environment, for example, are much weaker. Campaigning in the context of the workplace is therefore especially important. As we have seen, several unions are now attempting to implement 'no carcinogens' agreements (see appendix 5 for NGA sample carcinogens agreement). If this were to be successful, and if the activities of unions in this area could be broadened, then hopefully the power of organised labour could be used in the campaign to achieve a concerted regulatory attack on cancer – both inside and outside the workplace.

Public participation and democratic control

It would be wrong, however, to assume that the establishment of a more rational regulatory system would – in itself – solve the cancer problem. We also need to be concerned about *who* does the regulating and by what criteria. Thus, we also need to fight for a system that includes wider public participation and access to information.

Expertise has, of course, a considerable role to play in the regulatory process and specialised knowledge and experience are of the utmost importance. However, there is, at present, an imbalance in the distribution of expertise. Mechanisms need to be created by which such expert knowledge can be made more easily available to unions and to the whole range of public interest groups – probably through some form of public funding. At present, scientific and technical expertise is usually bought by the highest bidder, making effective intervention in the regulatory system difficult for affected individuals and groups with few resources. It is important to recognise that other people – 'non-experts', in the technical sense – also need to be involved in the regulatory process. The question of whether a carcinogen should be tolerated in the workplace, for instance, must be seen not merely as a technical question but as an important social and political issue because risk-takers *themselves* must decide if the risk is acceptable. It is vital, therefore, that we find some mechanism by which to enfranchise those groups and individuals who have something to contribute, but who cannot participate in the regulatory process as it stands. While informed and concerned members of the public or their representatives may at present give evidence to *some* of the various committees, they are not usually given the right to participate in the decision-making and it is this that needs to be changed.

Political pressure from the trade union movement has meant that they now have some say in certain decisions made in relation to the workplace. We need to increase this newly won participation and extend it to all other areas of the regulation of carcinogens. There are many possible models for such participation, but whatever the form and degree of 'non-specialist' participation we are able to achieve, it is vital that all those people involved in the regulatory process should be democratically accountable for their actions. Decisions should no longer be taken behind closed doors, and both the decisions themselves and the basis upon which they have been made must be open to public scrutiny – including the probing of conflicts of interests in members of expert advisory committees.

The process could begin with the publication of interim findings, plus the evidence and arguments used to arrive at these conclusions, by all of the current expert committees – PSPS, FACC, ACTS, etc. Comments from scientific peer groups and interested parties would be invited, and public hearings held on the main issues at stake some months later, under the auspices of the regulating government department. A right of final appeal could be vested in a multi-disciplinary council of scientists and citizens, independent of any one government department; nominations to the council would come from unions, consumer groups, employers, academia and the government. Such a council, though confined to scientists, has recently been proposed in Canada.[7] This more open and democratic procedure, which would have to be accompanied by a Freedom of Information Act, would be time- and resource-consuming. However, some emergency (but temporary) regulatory action could be taken to allow swift action on the side of caution whenever new evidence demanded it.

Finally, it is important that the regulatory system include some more open and democratic mechanism for the evaluation of the social usefulness of a chemical or product. Manufacturers developing new products are concerned primarily with profitability, rather than the true social usefulness of a material. The evaluation of any hazard only comes afterwards – often when the product is already on the market. We therefore need to push for a system which would ensure that the development of new products was carried out in the light both of their known or potential hazards and also of their social utility. The approval schemes for both drugs and food already contain this additional criterion – in principle, at least – and this test of social utility should be extended to the regulation of other types of chemicals. It is vital, however, that this determination of potential usefulness be made in an open and democratic manner.

Freedom of information and access to knowledge
But, in order to ensure the effectiveness of any regulatory system, two further conditions need to be met. First, more information of a different kind needs to be gathered about the incidence and causes of cancer. Second, this information, along with the data that already exist, must be opened up to public scrutiny, and made available *as a right* to anyone requesting it.

There is a pressing need for a more effective monitoring system, designed explicitly to look at patterns of health, sickness and death in the population as a whole. Such a system would represent an important advance on the present situation, where we remain largely dependent on partial information extracted from statistics designed for quite different purposes – birth and death certificates or hospital in-patient studies, for instance.[8] A system of this kind could greatly extend the usefulness of the information now obtained through the cancer registration scheme if it were designed to make possible the tracking of individuals through different jobs and places of residence. In this way, links could be made between possible occupational or environmental exposure and eventual ill-health or death. Record linkage between different government departments would obviously be of value here in trying to make such connections, but all companies should also be required to keep health records of employees and of their exposures, and to retain these for at least 40 years or until death. In addition, each factory should be required to keep a detailed register of materials used, and their quantities and where a worker had been exposed to a known carcinogen, this would be entered on the medical record kept by his/her GP. Obviously, there would be serious problems of confidentiality if any scheme of this kind were to be set up – the privacy of individuals would need to be guaranteed and this might prove difficult to achieve. Nevertheless, detailed record-keeping of this kind is essential, both to ensure compensation for individuals contracting cancer as a result of preventable exposure to carcinogens and to prevent future exposures. More fundamentally, it could play an essential part in the identification and ultimate elimination of avoidable cancers.

However, information is not in itself enough. It must also be freely available, and in a 'secretive' country like Britain, gaining access to such knowledge presents very serious problems. Britain still has no Freedom of Information Act of the kind found both in the USA and in several European countries.[9] On the contrary, all official information is assumed to be secret unless its release is specifically authorised. Indeed, anyone who does reveal or receive such information without authorisation is liable to a prison sentence under the Official Secrets Act of 1911. This legislation is at present used most effectively to keep civil servants at all levels quiet about matters of public concern – including those relating to health and safety. It is also used, along with Britain's stringent libel laws, to limit the degree of exposure such issues receive in the media. As an exception to this general rule, a few pieces of recent legislation have included specific provisions for the public disclosure of information – the Health and Safety at Work Act and the 1974 Control of Pollution Act being particularly relevant to the cancer issue.[10] However, these powers of disclosure have been only vaguely defined and are given to the Factory Inspectorate or the relevant local authority, rather than to individuals and groups. As a result, they have been very little used. Even the parliamentary commissioner or ombudsman, to whom citizens can complain about certain forms of maladministration, is subject to the same laws of secrecy and cannot reveal any findings unless permitted to do so by the relevant government departments.

Secrecy is widespread and even taken for granted in most areas of British administrative and political life. This has obvious implications for any campaign against cancer. A great deal of information about known or suspected carcinogens and their use comes into government hands through the functioning of the various regulatory authorities. However, this information is rarely passed on to the general public and hence cannot be used in preventive campaigns The Department of Employment, for instance, has recently admitted that hundreds of workers are not being informed that their X-rays show early signs of asbestosis.[11] At a local community level, Derbyshire County Council recently refused to reveal the siting of a new dump for highly toxic wastes.[12] It is important then that any campaign for cancer prevention must ally itself with the growing number of individuals and groups in Britain who have been fighting since the early 1970s for the introduction of a Freedom of Information Act. The open dissemination of information is a prerequisite for success in fighting against cancer, and this can only be achieved by breaking the virtual monopoly of industry and government over the relevant data.

Legal initiatives

We have seen, then, that the law as presently formulated gives very little help indeed to those wishing to get access to information. But can legal avenues be used in other ways in the fight against cancer? We have already seen in our discussion of the regulatory process that the access of cancer victims to the courts is extremely limited, both because of the high cost in terms of time and money, and also because English law rarely allows for 'class suits', so that the full responsibility for any action has to be borne by the victim alone. In addition, for a compensation case to be successful, workers have to prove employer's negligence *as well as* 'cause and effect'. Radiation is the only exception where cause and effect alone needs to be established. Since cancers usually take many years both to become apparent and also to become associated with particular substances, it is frequently impossible to prove negligence by employers. When the cancer victims themselves provide the first 'acceptable' evidence that a substance causes cancer, how can the employer's behaviour of 20 years ago be held to be negligent? This provides one more reason why non-human data alone (animal or mutagenicity tests) should be regarded as sufficient for preventive action. In the meantime, several unions are now demanding 'no fault' compensation schemes for all occupational diseases.

While unions are continuing to support certain of their members in compensation cases, the use of the law by individuals and groups to fight cases of exposure to carcinogenic or other toxic substances occurring *outside* the workplace has been rare and notoriously difficult. This is well illustrated by a recent case in which three London parents attempted to sue the oil companies at common law for the neurological damage they alleged that lead additives in petrol had done to their children.[13] This was finally quashed in the High Court by a judge who ruled that the companies had no case to answer. This was two years after the suit had been filed. Had the parents taken the case further, to the House of Lords – *just for the right to have their claims heard* – it might have dragged on for several more years, exhausting and bankrupting the claimants.

Conclusion

We have shown that individuals can take some action to reduce their own exposure to carcinogens. However, we have also demonstrated that individual actions of this kind are not enough, and have outlined the most basic elements that need to be considered in a more broadly based campaign against cancer. Such a campaign should have *eight basic demands*.

1 Britain should have a 'generic' cancer policy for the identification, assessment and control of potential carcinogens

both inside and outside the workplace, rather than the fragmented and partial approach that currently operates.

2 An adequately funded and democratically accountable institute should be set up, independent of corporate control, for the testing and evaluation of toxic materials and for toxicological research.

3 Much greater emphasis needs to be placed on cancer prevention by the cancer charities and by government research institutes. There should be an increase in the funding of toxicological and epidemiological research, on cancer causation and an emphasis on the examination of the effects of occupational and environmental factors on different social groups.

4 A list of all known and suspected carcinogens and associated safety precautions should be issued and all products properly labelled.

5 There should be a Freedom of Information Act to allow greater public knowledge of scientific and medical information on carcinogens and how they are used. This should apply to information produced by private and public corporations and by regulatory authorities.

6 There must be public participation and openness in decision-making over control of carcinogenic substances with the active involvement of all interest groups likely to be affected. Advisory bodies should be set up on a representative rather than a purely 'expert' basis and groups involved in such bodies should have state funds made available to ensure their effective participation.

7 New criteria for social utility need to be established. There should be greater public discussion of the criteria by which the risks of a suspected carcinogen and its potential social usefulness can be judged. To start the process, regulatory authorities should specify the procedures whereby they currently make their assessments.

8 There should be a stronger anti-smoking campaign, involving the banning of advertising and promotion of all smoking materials, the provision of increased counselling facilities for smokers, the banning of smoking in public places (including

workplaces), a long-term plan for the redeployment of workers dependent on tobacco processing, distribution and sale, and assistance for third world governments who wish to restrict the growing use of tobacco in their countries but are not able to counter the economic power of the tobacco multinationals.

These, then, are the basic elements in an anti-cancer campaign. However, it is important to stress at the outset that the struggle will not be easy. In making demands of this kind we are not merely demanding narrowly based administrative or regulatory reform, but fundamental changes in how decisions are made in our society. In so doing, we will inevitably confront extremely powerful groups who have a vested interest in maintaining the system essentially as it is – even though people will continue to die unnecessarily of cancer. Moreover, the basic problem is not the immoral and self-serving behaviour of individual firms, the bureaucratic inefficiency of government agencies or the disinterest or capture of certain sections of the scientific establishment. The problem is inherent in the nature and priorities of a society in which the profit motive is predominant. Indeed, the fight against cancer is inextricably linked to the need to deal with the most basic injustices and inequalities of industrial capitalism. We cannot separate the struggle to save ourselves and others from cancer from the fight to create a society in which human needs rank higher than commercial interests.

Appendices

Appendix 1. Evaluation of carcinogenicity of chemicals and occupational groups at risk

Chemicals or industrial processes associated with cancer induction in humans: comparison of target organs and main routes of exposure in animals and humans*

| Chemical or industrial process | Humans | | |
	Main type of exposure[a]	Target organ	Main route of exposure[b]
1. Aflatoxins	Environmental, occupational[c]	Liver	p.o., inhalation[c]
2. 4-Aminobiphenyl	Occupational	Bladder	Inhalation, skin, p.o.
3. Arsenic compounds	Occupational, medicinal, and environmental	Skin, lung, liver[c]	Inhalation, p.o., skin

* *(Source* L. Tomatis *et al., Cancer Research,* vol. 38 (1978), pp. 877–85); see also IARC Monograph Supplement 4, *Chemicals, Industrial Processes and Industries Associated with Cancer in Humans*, IARC, Lyon, France, 1982.

	Animals	
Animal	Target organ	Route of exposure
Rat	Liver, stomach, colon, kidney	p.o.
Fish, duck, marmoset, tree shrew, monkey	Liver	p.o.
Rat	Liver, trachea	i.t.
	Liver	i.p.
Mouse, rat	Local	s.c. injection
Mouse	Lung	i.p.
Mouse, rabbit, dog	Bladder	p.o.
Newborn mouse	Liver	s.c. injection
Rat	Mammary gland, intestine	s.c. injection
Mouse, rat, dog	Inadequate, negative	p.o.
Mouse	Inadequate, negative	Topical, i.v.

| Chemical or industrial process | Humans | | |
	Main type of exposure[a]	Target organ	Main route of exposure[b]
4. Asbestos	Occupational	Lung, pleural cavity, gastro-intestinal tract	Inhalation, p.o.
5. Auramine (manufacture of)	Occupational	Bladder	Inhalation, skin, p.o.
6. Benzene	Occupational	Haemopoietic system	Inhalation, skin
7. Benzidine	Occupational	Bladder	Inhalation, skin, p.o.
8. Bis(chloromethyl) ether	Occupational	Lung	Inhalation
9. Cadmium-using industries (possibly cadmium oxide)	Occupational	Prostate, lung[c]	Inhalation, p.o.
10. Chloramphenicol	Medicinal	Haemopoietic system	p.o., injection
11. Chloromethyl methyl ether (possibly associated with bis(chloromethyl) ether)	Occupational	Lung	Inhalation

Animal	Animals	
	Target organ	Route of exposure
Mouse, rat, hamster, rabbit	Lung, pleura	Inhalation or i.t.
Rat, hamster	Local	Intrapleural
Rat	Local	i.p., s.c. injection
	Various sites[c]	p.o.
Mouse, rat	Liver	p.o.
Rabbit, dog	Negative	p.o.
Rat	Local, liver, intestine	s.c. injection
Mouse	Inadequate	Topical, s.c. injection
Mouse	Liver	s.c. injection
Rat	Liver	p.o.
	Zymbal gland, liver, colon	s.c. injection
Hamster	Liver	p.o.
Dog	Bladder	p.o.
Mouse, rat	Lung, nasal cavity	Inhalation
Mouse	Skin	Topical
	Local, lung	s.c. injection
Rat	Local	s.c. injection
Rat	Local, testis	s.c. or i.m. injection
	No adequate tests	
Mouse	Initiator	Skin
	Lung[c]	Inhalation
	Local, lung[c]	s.c. injection
Rat	Local[c]	s.c. injection

Chemical or industrial process	Humans		
	Main type of exposure[a]	Target organ	Main route of exposure[b]
12. Chromium (chromate-producing industries)	Occupational	Lung, nasal cavities[c]	Inhalation
13. Cyclophosphamide	Medicinal	Bladder	p.o., injection
14. Diethylstilboestrol	Medicinal	Uterus, vagina	p.o.
15. Hematite mining (? radon)	Occupational	Lung	Inhalation
16. Isopropyl oils	Occupational	Nasal cavity, larynx	Inhalation
17. Melphalan	Medicinal	Haemopoietic system	p.o., injection
18. Mustard gas	Occupational	Lung, larynx	Inhalation

Animal	Animals Target organ	Route of exposure
Mouse, rat	Local	s.c., i.m. injection
Rat	Lung	Intrabronchial implantation
Mouse	Haemopoietic system, lung	i.p., s.c. injection
	Various sites	p.o.
Rat	Bladder[c]	i.p.
	Mammary gland	i.p.
	Various sites	i.v.
Mouse	Mammary	p.o.
Mouse	Mammary, lymphoreticular testis	s.c. injection, s.c. implantation
	vagina	Local
Rat	Mammary, hypophysis[c] bladder	s.c. implantation
Hamster	Kidney	s.c. injection, s.c. implantation
Squirrel monkey	Uterine serosa	s.c. implantation
Mouse, hamster, guinea pig	Negative	Inhalation, i.t.
Rat	Negative	s.c. injection
	No adequate tests	
Mouse	Initiator	Skin
	Lung, lympho- sarcomas	i.p.
Rat	Local	i.p.
Mouse	Lung	Inhalation, i.v.
	Local, mammary	s.c. injection

| Chemical or industrial process | Humans | | |
	Main type of exposure[a]	Target organ	Main route of exposure[b]
19. 2-Naphthylamine	Occupational	Bladder	Inhalation, skin, p.o.
20. Nickel (nickel refining)	Occupational	Nasal cavity, lung	Inhalation
21. N,N-Bis(2-chloroethyl)-2-naphthylamine	Medicinal	Bladder	p.o
22. Oxymetholone	Medicinal	Liver	p.o.
23. Phenacetin	Medicinal	Kidney	p.o.
24. Phenytoin	Medicinal	Lymphoreticular tissues	p.o., injection
25. Soot, tars, and oils	Occupational, environmental	Lung, skin (scrotum)	Inhalation, skin
26. Vinyl chloride	Occupational	Liver, brain,[c] lung[c]	Inhalation, skin

	Animals	
Animal	Target organ	Route of exposure
Hamster, dog, monkey	Bladder	p.o.
Mouse	Liver, lung	s.c. injection
Rat, rabbit	Inadequate	p.o.
Rat	Lung	Inhalation,
Mouse, rat, hamster	Local	s.c., i.m. injection
Mouse, rat	Local	i.m. implantation
Mouse	Lung	i.p.
Rat	Local	s.c. injection
	No adequate tests	
	No adequate tests[d]	
Mouse	Lymphoreticular tissues	p.o., i.p.
Mouse, rabbit	Skin	Topical
Mouse, rat	Lung, liver, blood vessels, mammary, Zymbal gland, Kidney	Inhalation

[a] The main types of exposures mentioned are those by which the association has been demonstrated; exposures other than those mentioned may also occur.

[b] The main routes of exposure given may not be the only ones by which such effects could occur.

[c] Indicative evidence.

[d] The induction of the nasal cavities in rats given phenacetin has been reported recently (S. Odashima, personal communication, 1977).

Abbreviations i.t. = intra tracheally (through the trachea); i.m. = intra muscularly; i.v. = intra venous; p.o. = per os (through the mouth); s.c. = subcutaneous (under the skin); i.p. = intra-peritoneally.

Occupational groups with increased cancer risk but no identified specific cause*

Epidemiological studies of a number of occupational groups have found that cancer levels in them are raised, although no particular cause to explain this has been identified. The following table lists most of the occupational groups in this category.

Occupational groups	Cancer site(s)
Coal miners	Stomach
Chemists	Pancreas, lymphomas
Chemical workers	Several
Foundry workers	Lung
Textile workers	Mouth and pharynx
Printing pressmen (newspapers)	Mouth and pharynx
Metal miners	Lung
Coke by-product workers	Large intestine, pancreas
Cadmium production workers	Prostate
Rubber industry	
Processing	Stomach, leukaemia
Tyre building	Bladder, brain
Tyre curing	Lung
Furniture workers**	Nasal cavity and sinuses
Shoe workers**	Nasal cavity and sinuses
	Leukaemia
Leather workers	Bladder

* This section reproduced from *Cancer and Work*, City University Statistical Laboratory and GMWU (1983).
** There is little doubt that the nasal cancers are of occupational origin but the cause is as yet unknown.

Appendix 2. Distorting the epidemiology of cancer: the need for a more balanced overview*
Richard Peto

There exist, both in the general environment and in certain occupations, chemical or physical agents which increase the likelihood of human cancer. Our political response to this would, in an ideal world where sufficient knowledge was available, depend on the direct and indirect costs of the various possible measures of control, and on how many cancers each such measure would prevent. In the real world, estimates of the direct financial costs of the control of particular agents can easily differ by one or two orders of magnitude, the indirect costs may be grossly exaggerated, or some major indirect costs may be completely overlooked. Worst of all, we have in general no remotely reliable estimates of the numbers of cancers which particular legislative controls would prevent. Consequently, there is wide scope for pressure groups to have considerable influence on public policy.

Historically, the most powerful pressure groups in US society have been the large financial interests, which have almost always put financial advantage before human health. Over the past few years the major tobacco companies have launched massive sales drives in the third world, which if successful will kill millions of people. (About one in four regular cigarette smokers is killed prematurely by smoking.) In the USA, where cigarettes cause well over 100,000 deaths every year from lung cancer or chronic obstructive lung disease, the tobacco industry refuses to accept in public that cigarettes cause either disease, let alone to collaborate in serious public information, and no epithet can suitably describe the collective efforts of their advertisers.

No other industry kills people on anything like the scale that the tobacco industry does, but where other industries have been found to cause cancer (or dust-induced lung disease) in their workers or in the

---

* This appendix originally appeared in *Nature*, vol. 284, 27 March 1980. It developed from a review of Samuel Epstein, *The Politics of Cancer*, Anchor Press (1979). Reproduced by permission from *Nature*, vol. 284 © 1980 Macmillan Journals Ltd.

consumers of their products, their immediate response has usually been to delay acceptance of the findings, to minimise their relevance to current practice, and in general to delay or obstruct any hygienic measures which will cost money. Even when human danger has been unequivocally demonstrated, industrial consortia may actively lobby for controls so weak that (as with the new UK government regulations limiting inhaled asbestos to 1 fibre/ml from 1981) they leave no reasonable safety margin. Large amounts of money are available to mount press or TV publicity campaigns about the homely apple-pie virtues of asbestos, journals financed by the tobacco industry run populist articles which misrepresent research results to lay readers, and some American television journalists are explicitly told always to censor all reference to the dangers of smoking.

Even the scientific literature is not immune from distortion by financial interests. The decades-long argument that 'threshold' dose levels of carcinogens must exist below which the general population is absolutely safe has not been entirely motivated by the scientific plausibility of the hypothesis. With increasing understanding of the derivation of tumours from single cells acted on by mutagenic carcinogens, industry is slowly abandoning 'threshold' arguments in favour of arguments[1,2] (where the biological fallacies[3,4] are somewhat better concealed by the mathematics) that thousandfold reductions in dose can conveniently be 'statistically guaranteed' to produce a millionfold or some other enormous reduction in risk.

Even if the scientists who propounded such models are disinterested, industrial endorsement of them is not. Much excellent toxicology may be done by industry, and many industrial scientists and managers may be directly and honestly concerned with the prevention of hazards. But so many examples of financially-motivated bias exist that the motives and work of industrial scientists and consultants are inevitably distrusted.

Over the past quarter century, the 'environmentalist' camp in North American society has pressed for (and achieved) stricter control of particular carcinogens in the workplace, the general environment, and the diet. Usually, their efforts have been directly resisted by the relevant financial interests. Inevitably, in view of the scantiness of reliable quantitative knowledge about the cancer risks to man of nearly all carcinogens, the argument has polarised. In the politics of cancer, each side takes a very extreme position. Industry usually argues for the irrelevance to man of animal or *in vitro* cancer tests, or minimises the quantitative hazards and exaggerates the costs of control. The environmentalists usually exaggerate the likely hazards and are largely indifferent to the costs of control. The vacuum of reliable scientific knowledge is such that each side can find scientists who will maintain in courts, in public hearings or in the scientific literature whatever is politically convenient, and it is important to recognise that scientists on both sides of this debate now have career interests at stake in it.

A particularly good example of the biased writings of politically active environmentalists is Samuel Epstein's *The Politics of Cancer* (Sierra Club Books, 1978, revised in Anchor Press, 1979). Epstein outlines, for university-educated but not necessarily science-educated readers, his view of our present state of knowledge about prevention of death from cancer. He concludes that the cure rates for the major cancers have not been improving much over recent years, but that we do know enough now about the causes of cancer for the testing and regulation of environmental contaminants to prevent the majority of American cancer deaths, and that the main obstacles to our doing so are political rather than scientific. He therefore reviews the scientific and political circumstances surrounding a dozen or so disputed consumer products or occupational hazards, providing much fascinating political detail, and then describes at length the internal politics of the various agencies which research, regulate and litigate in Washington.

Epstein's book has been written to inflame political passions against environmental carcinogens, and parts of it are well worth reading. However, the political punch is often achieved at the expense of scientific accuracy and balance. Despite this, the book has already gained wide and apparently uncritical acceptance even among scientists. For that reason, it is worth considering some of the misrepresentations of scientific evidence which it contains, and some of the more general defects in the environmentalist perspective on cancer.

First, a few details. Epstein's book is very useful as a source of reference to original papers, but it is not in itself a reliable secondary reference because the material presented is so often distorted. Sometimes this distortion is due to the effects of Epstein's vigorous campaigning style on his scientific judgement and is, perhaps, forgivable; at other times it appears to be deliberate, which cannot so easily be forgiven.

For example, consider the (by now generally agreed) finding that incorporation of about 5 per cent by weight of saccharin into rat diets gives a few rats bladder cancer, but has no generally accepted effects on any other type of cancer. By human standards, 5 per cent represents a vast saccharin intake (and so, of course, the industrial 'Calorie Control Council' have tried to shrug off these findings). To refute the common reaction that 'anything given in large enough doses will cause cancer in animals', Epstein's chief argument is to report that 0.01 per cent saccharin has also been shown to be carcinogenic. In support of this extraordinary claim, he presents in tabular form the control and 0.01 per cent data for

Table A.1 Data from OTA report[5] on the tumour sites selected for presentation in Epstein's book to subtantiate the claim that 0.01 per cent saccharin is carcinogenic. Groups selectively omitted in Epstein's book are marked with an asterisk. These omissions substantially alter the implications of the original data

Saccharin dose (% in rat diet; these doses have no material effect on longevity)	Male or female lymphosarcomas (FDA, 1948)	Female breast (FDA, 1973)	Male breast (FDA, 1973)
0 (control)	0/20[+] (0%)	6/26 (23%)	6/29 (21%)
0.01	8/14 (57%)	14/30 (47%)	14/25 (56%)
0.1	5/16 (31%)*	13/34 (38%)*	9/27 (33%)*
0.5	2/15 (13%)*	—	—
1	1/18 (6%)*	12/30 (40%)*	8/27 (30%)*
5	10/17 (59%)	12/27 (44%)*	7/25 (28%)*

* Omitted in Epstein's book.
† In addition to these 20, since some other sweeteners were being tested concurrently, 34 other control animals were studied in the same experiment, and the 1977 OTA review of these data, considering all the control animals to be equivalent, cited 9/54 control lymphosarcomas. (0/10 saccharin controls of each sex were studied, not 0/20 as Epstein inadvertently indicated.)

selected cancers from certain multi-group feeding experiments, leaving out the observations from those same experiments which would have refuted it (see table A.1). This appears to be a deliberate attempt to deceive the reader. It is not a casual slip in a 600-page book, as Epstein devotes twenty pages and two full-page tables to saccharin. His entire table 6.4, entitled 'Tumours other than the bladder in rodents fed saccharin', appears to be so subject to artefacts of selection that it provides no evidence that saccharin does cause any rodent tumours other than in the rat bladder.

Saccharin is not an isolated example of bias; indeed, I found that in many places where he discussed data with which I was familiar inaccuracies were present, almost always in the direction of accentuating the need for battle with the devils of industry.

Turning to more important matters, Epstein asserts that any benefits from the 'less dangerous' cigarettes which the tobacco industry has developed will be outweighed by people increasing their consumption to get more nicotine, and he is therefore in many places particularly scathing about (or even downright opposed to) research into changed cigarette composition. This is a distorted perspective on one of the more promising

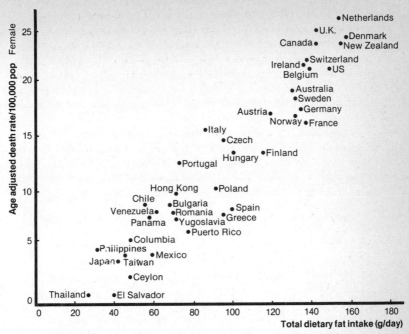

Figure A.1 Data[9] plotting for 39 countries age-adjusted breast cancer death rate versus dietary fat intake (animal or vegetable).

immediate means of preventing fatal cancers, a quarter of which in America are currently due to smoking.

Smokers of 'less dangerous' cigarettes have already been found in various epidemiological studies to have disease rates which are materially lower than smokers of other cigarettes;[6, 7] at autopsy they have far fewer 'pre-malignant' histological changes in their bronchi[8] and, perhaps due to the changes in cigarette composition 10 or 20 years ago male lung cancer death rates in early middle age are now decreasing in North America, in Britain and in Finland.[9]

After lung, the next commonest fatal cancers in the USA are those of the breast and the large intestine, for which the most striking epidemiological finding to date is a 90 per cent correlation between fat consumption in different countries and their breast or colon cancer rates (see figure A.1; similar correlations exist for colon cancer).[10] Epstein suggests that dietary fat may merely be acting as a vehicle for fat-soluble pesticides and industrial chemicals, which predictably emerge as his villains yet again. However, his suggestion is implausible: countries with high levels of contamination do not stand out from the general cancer/fat relationship, colorectal and breast cancer were common long before the widespread use of pesticides, and in experimental animals high-fat or low-fat diets can greatly enhance or reduce the risk of cancer.[11] Something more interesting is waiting to be discovered in our diet than simple contamination by carcinogens.

The fat-associated and smoking-derived cancers collectively account for more than half of all cancer deaths, and people concerned with cancer politics should try to understand them considerably more accurately than Epstein appears to. One can list many other instances where Epstein's content or style are misleading or unbalanced. For example:

- The discussion of alcoholism and cancer is entirely erroneous because of failure to standardise properly for age.
- One of Epstein's chapters ends: 'Eisenhower warned against the growing national threat of the military-industrial complex. The medical-industrial complex now appears to be as serious a threat.'
- There is idealisation of the value of long-term animal tests with concomitant denigration of the value of the Ames test and other short-term tests. This is one of Epstein's most inexplicable errors of scientific judgement, unless he wants cancer tests to be difficult and expensive for industry.
- He is irritatingly puritanical, sneering at 'the plastic age which symbolises how the value of our life-style has been degraded'.
- He seeks by stylistic tricks to attribute to oral contraceptives some of the established hazards of hormone replacement therapy and of diethylstilboestrol.
- He claims that cancer costs the American economy over $25 billion per year. (In fact, cancer must be prevented for humane, not for economic reasons; without cancer, there would be three or four million more retired North Americans to support, costing over $25 billion per year).

And so on. He seems so certain about everything – how can anybody be justified in being so certain about so many details? Sometimes I know he's wrong, but more often (especially in the many places where inconclusive scientific results are presented as established fact) I know that nobody knows for sure. Lewis Thomas once wrote, in another context:

> The sceptics in medicine have a hard time of it. It is much more difficult to be convincing about ignorance concerning disease

mechanisms than it is to make claims for full comprehension, especially when the comprehension leads, logically or not, to some sort of action. When it comes to serious illness, the public tends, understandably, to be more sceptical about the sceptics, more willing to believe the true believers.

Epstein (like many others) is unjustifiably definite about three major issues. He seems certain that even after the effects of cigarettes have been allowed for, Americans live in an era of rapidly increasing cancer rates. But trends in recorded cancer death rates (and, perhaps more so, recorded incidence rates) over the past quarter century are biased upwards (since the cure rates for the major cancers have not materially improved) by improvements in medical care and cancer counting. These improvements have affected all sectors of US society, but most particularly old people and previously poor people, especially blacks. Epstein, along with most other American commentators, does not allow for these biases even to the limited extent of restricting his attention to trends in age-specific mortality rates among middle-aged whites, where they might be expected to be least prominent.

Among middle-aged whites during the past quarter century, cancer cure rates have not materially improved, but some US cancer mortality trends seem to be genuinely down (stomach, cervix) while some seem to be genuinely up (pancreas, melanoma, and certain lymphomas). I can discern no net pattern other than that due to the massive effects of smoking on lung cancer, although no extension to 1978 yet exists of the excellent 1950–67 trend analyses in NCI monograph 33. In Britain, the same is true[12] as long as we examine mortality in middle age. (Interestingly, although Epstein emphasises that bladder cancer death rates among whites in the industrial north-eastern USA are high, this may not be chiefly due to any current industrial hazard, for they have been decreasing both relatively and absolutely for a quarter of a century.)[13]

Epstein also seems certain that the majority of human cancer is caused by chemical and physical agents in the environment and could be prevented by their testing and regulation. There is no sound scientific basis for this certainty. Since the cancers (lung, breast, large intestine) which are commonest in the USA are rare in certain other countries, and *vice versa*, they probably really are preventable, but (see figure A.1) not necessarily by regulation of any environmental pollutants or food additives. Indeed, one of the most intriguing animal findings is the effect in many studies of gross aspects of diet on cancer; for example, mice randomised between 5g of food once daily and *ad lib* consumption averaging 6g/day of the same food, had respectively 8 per cent and 64 per cent spontaneous mammary tumours,[14] and the role of dietary fat[11] has already been discussed.

Thirdly, Epstein seems certain that at least a quarter of all cancer deaths are attributable to occupational exposure to carcinogens. There is as yet no good evidence for hazards of anything like this magnitude, and there is clear evidence that many of his particular claims are exaggerated. For example, he says that asbestos has led to approximately 50,000 deaths per year in the USA from cancer and related disease (referencing a paper by Selikoff[15] which actually neither makes nor implies any such claim). This is sheer nonsense; of 50,000 asbestos deaths, several thousand should be certified as being due to pleural mesothelioma, yet only several hundred per year are thus certified.

Likewise, Epstein cites with approval (indeed, he describes it as being of 'epochal significance') Health, Education and Welfare Secretary Califano's absurd 1978 estimate, in a speech to labour union leaders, that as many as half of the 8–11 million workers who have been exposed to asbestos could develop serious diseases such as cancer or asbestosis. In his second edition, Epstein draws extensively on Califano's source, a curious but extremely influential document which has been circulating privately for the past year or more. This unpublished typescript, with no listed authors, was prepared by a working group of nine well-known scientists including Arthur Upton and David Rall, the National Cancer Institute and National Institute of Environmental Health Sciences directors, both of whom still seem more ready to defend than to repudiate it.

Entitled 'Estimates of the fraction of cancer in the US related to occupational factors', it shows how a group of reasonable men can collectively generate an unreasonable report. The group multiplied the 12 million workers exposed in any way in 1972–4 to any of asbestos, As, Ni, Cr, benzene or petrochemicals by the very large risk factors (e.g. fivefold lung cancer excesses) typical of much more extensively exposed industrial populations, finally multiplying again by '4–5' to allow for the additional cancers that will be caused by these six agents among workers exposed to them at times other than 1972–4. (In casual disregard of dosimetry, this whole process is very like predicting 100,000 occupational lung cancer deaths per year among non-smokers due to their exposure to other people's cigarette smoke at work, 'since 20 per cent of heavy smokers get lung cancer'.)

These assumptions 'predict' over 200,000 extra respiratory tract cancers per year in the near future due to the above six agents alone (and are the sole source of the currently widespread prediction of '20–30 per cent' of cancers being due to occupation). But, in reality, fewer than 90,000 males/year get respiratory tract cancer in the US (and most of these are due to cigarettes and not to occupation at all) and moreover the USA male rates in the first 25 years of working life are currently decreasing! A prediction of 100,000–200,000 extras due to the above six agents is clearly very unrealistic.

The unreality of the whole method is further highlighted by the fact that the assumptions 'predict' $7,300 \times 4.5$ nickel-oxide induced occupational lung cancers/year. Since nickel refining causes a lot of nasal as well as lung cancer, we would presumably then also soon 'expect' something like 13,000 nasal cancer death certificates per year among nickel workers. Nickel has already been widely used for decades, so many thousands of these should presumably already be evident. In reality, each year in the American population there are only 300-odd male and 200-odd female nasal cancer death certificates. The majority of these are not ex-nickel workers and no marked trends are evident. This demonstrates the unsoundness of the NCI-NIEHS methodology.

Unfortunately, such exaggerated estimates are so much what many people want to believe of modern society that they have now achieved a life of their own, and although they are utterly without foundation they are quoted widely, repeatedly and reputably both in the lay and scientific press. In Geneva the International Labour Organisation reportedly endorsed them, as did the Toxic Substances Strategy Committee in their recent draft report to the American president,[16] and they have been used in OSHA to emphasise the need for stricter laws. Most recently, the British trade union the Association of Scientific, Technical and Managerial Staffs (ASTMS) released a policy document which appears to have been strongly influened by Epstein's book, and which is notable for its prominent but erroneous assertion, derived solely from the foregoing unpublished American typescript, that 20–40 per cent of current British cancer deaths are caused by occupational carcinogens.

Epstein now claims that these exaggerated estimates seriously underestimate the impact of industrial carcinogens. There is obviously a valid political need to exaggerate the importance of the preventive measures we can already implement, but in the long run we do also still need to discover the main preventable causes of cancer other than smoking. Bearing both these needs in mind, there are limits beyond which it is not even politically wise to distort the science of cancer, and some of today's exaggerations may well transgress those limits. Reliable reviews of the known and suspected causes[17, 18, 19] of human cancer and of trends in British death rates[12] should be more widely known.

My criticisms of Epstein's science, however, must be viewed in the light of the continued resistance of many industries to reasonable controls. One has only to read some of his descriptions of industrial behaviour to see where his passion comes from, and a suitably sceptical reader could derive much important information from the dozen or so detailed case-histories of particular carcinogens that make up the bulk of this book. But, although I cannot prove it, I suspect that environmentalists as a whole (including Epstein and those US and British trade unions which have already modelled their public statements closely on his book) would be better respected and could therefore press more effectively for controls in particular instances if their overview of cancer was more balanced in the following ways:

- if they accepted that present-day cancer rates and trends are probably not dominated by occupational carcinogens or environmental pollutants (especially since they could still warn that future rates might perhaps be so dominated unless present-day exposures are regulated[20]);
- if their chief concern was with the identification and control of the few major determinants of human cancer (or, in an industrial context, the few major industrial carcinogens) rather than the large multitude of sins which Epstein denounces;
- if they discussed the costs and benefits of research into the control of toxic substances in the context of other possible ways of improving longevity (bad diet and tobacco in rich countries, malnutrition and infective and parasitic diseases elsewhere);
- if they took the costs of imposing restrictions on society more seriously. Epstein's general assertion is that the total direct and indirect costs of failing to regulate usually exceed the real costs of the testing and regulation, but I suspect that this is a slogan to avoid political embarrassment rather than a carefully researched conclusion;
- if they accepted that for most toxic chemicals we have both qualitative and vast quantitative uncertainty about the health benefits of restriction.

Particularly, even if the sort of grossly biased interpretation which Epstein applied to the animal saccharin data is avoided, the results of animal experiments simply are not an uncomplicated key to human hazard identification. First, moderate alteration of gross aspects of the diet of animals greatly modifies their spontaneous tumour onset rates[11] (so, for example, increasing the sugar content of rat diets may increase their cancer rates more than the equivalent amount of dietary saccharin would have done[11]). Also any chemical which causes proliferation or necrosis in any organ that is subject to spontaneous cancers is likely to modify the onset rate of tumours in that organ, and since the aim of most animal experiments is to study a dose which is nearly, but not quite, sufficient to cause significant weight loss or mortality within three months, it is not surprising that so many chemicals at such doses can cause cancer in animals.

However, it may be that where adversary politics operate one needs views at both extremes in order to get a balanced outcome. And there is a possibility that over-emphasis on the avoidance of scientific error would emasculate the environmentalist passions and merely lead to my own rather inactive conservatism. (After all, no scruples about scientific certainty of safety usually precede the widespread introduction of new chemicals, so should the imposition of prudent restrictions require absolute proof?)

Environmentalists with biased judgements and a quasireligious certainty of right will fight more battles than any reasonable sceptic would do, and even if their victories confer 10 or 100 times less benefit on humanity than they imagine, they will in the long run probably do more good than harm – unless they materially reduce food production, distort research priorities, or direct attention away from the smoking problem in the process. Epstein justly quotes, from the 1st century AD, the Plutarch chronicles: 'He who in time of faction takes neither side shall be disenfranchised'. So, I feel, should both environmentalists and industrialists who suppress or deliberately misinterpret data, but they probably won't be. For the moment, the 'politics of cancer' is dominated on both sides by exaggeration.

Notes

1. Cornfield, J. *Science* **198**, 693 (1977).
2. Mantel, N. and Schneidermann, M. A. *Cancer Research* **35**, 1379 (1975).
3. Crump, K. S. *et al., Cancer Research* **36**, 2973 (1976).
4. Guess, W. A. *et al., Cancer Research* **37**, 3475 (1977).
5. Office of Technology Assessment of the US Congress (1977): *Cancer Testing Technology and Saccharin.*
6. Hammond, E. C. *et al.,* in *Origins of Human Cancer*, Cold Spring Harbor NY (1977).
7. Wynder, E. L. *et al.,* in US government DHEW publication NIH 76-1221 (1976).
8. Auerbach, O. *et al., N.Engl.J.Med.* **300**, 381 (1979).
9. Caroll, K. K. *Cancer Research* **35**, 3374 (1975).
10. Armstrong, B. K. and Doll, R. *Int.J.Cancer* **15**, 617 (1975).

11. Jose, D. G. *Nutrition and Cancer* **1(3)**, 58 (1979). (Many other papers in all the 1979 issues of this journal are of great general interest e.g. **1(3)** 35, 67 and 27. See also part 2 of November 1975 *Cancer Research* devoted wholly to mutation and cancer).
12. Doll, R. *Proc.Roy.Soc.Lond.(B)* **205**, 47 (1979).
13. Blot, W. J. and Fraumeni, J. F. *Natl.Cancer Inst.* **61**, 1017 (1978).
14. Roe, F. J. C. and Tucker, M. J. *Excerpta Medica* (Int. Congress Series) **311**, 171 (1974).
15. Selikoff, I. J. in 'Origins of Human Cancer', Cold Spring Harbor NY (1977).
16. Norman, A. *Nature* **280**, 623 (1979).
17. Doll, R. *Nature* **265**, 589 (1977).
18. Doll, R. *Nutrition and Cancer* **1(3)**, 35 (1979).
19. IARC working group *Cancer Research* **40**, 1 (1980).
20. Davis, D. L. and Magee, B. H. *Science* **206**, 1356 (1979).

Appendix 3. Fallacies of life-style cancer theories*
Samuel S. Epstein and Joel B. Swartz

Peto's article,[1] purporting to be a review of the book *The Politics of Cancer*,[2] is largely a restatement of the lifestyle theory of cancer causation. This theory postulates that if you get cancer it is essentially your own fault, and that the causal role of past involuntary exposure to environmental and occupational carcinogens is trivial. Not surprisingly, the lifestyle theory has emerged as the major professed basis of the chemical industry's objections to the regulation of its carcinogenic products and processes.[3] As an enthusiastic proponent of this theory, Peto asserts that smoking-derived and fat-associated cancers 'collectively account for more than half of all cancer deaths.' As a corollary of Peto's emphasis on lifestyle factors, he denigrates the role of occupational and environmental carcinogens and the need for their effective regulation, claiming that there has been no recent increase in cancer mortality rates other than that due to smoking. We shall demonstrate that there is scant scientific basis for the lifestyle theory, and that it is in fact contradicted by a substantial body of published evidence.

Cancer rate trends

Peto justifies his emphasis on lifestyle factors by dismissing evidence for recently increasing cancer rates, apart from 'that due to the massive effects of smoking on lung cancer'. However, there is substantial evidence to the contrary. Standardised cancer death rates, adjusted to the 1940 age structure of the total United States population, show a progressive overall increase of about 7 per cent from 1935 to 1970[4] despite marked reductions of stomach cancer rates for unexplained reasons and of cervix cancer rates for reasons including the frequency of elective hysterectomy for non-malignant disease and the success of screening programmes. These trends are consistent with standardised mortality data for the

---

* This appendix originally appeared in *Nature*, vol. 289, 15 January 1981.
  Reproduced by permission from *Nature*, vol. 289 © 1981 Macmillan Journals Ltd.

United States (table A.2),[5] where they are even more marked in black males, and with crude mortality data for the United Kingdom (table A.3).[6] The overall rate of increase in US cancer mortality in the 7-year period from 1969 to 1976 (5.5 per cent), adjusted to the 1970 age structure,

Table A.2 Age-adjusted cancer mortality rates per 100,000 US population for selected sites by sex and year 1969–76, and average per cent change[5]

Site	Sex*	Mortality rate per 100,000		Average % change 1969–76	
		1969	1976	Annual	7-Year
All sites	WM	195.0	210.2	0.9	7.8
	WF	129.0	133.8	0.5	3.7
Stomach	WM	10.6	8.7	−2.9	−17.4
	WF	5.3	4.1	−3.6	−22.6
Colon	WM	18.7	20.7	1.3	10.7
	WF	16.2	16.5	0.0	1.9
Rectum	WM	6.9	5.6	−3.0	−18.8
	WF	3.9	3.2	−3.1	−17.9
Pancreas	WM	11.0	11.0	0.0	0.0
	WF	6.6	6.8	0.3	3.0
Lung	WM	55.0	66.7	2.6	21.3
	WF	10.2	17.8	7.6	74.5
Melanoma	WM	2.0	2.6	4.0	30.0
	WF	1.4	1.6	0.8	14.3
Breast	WF	26.2	27.2	0.3	3.8
Cervix	WF	5.5	3.9	−4.9	−29.1
Uterus	WF	4.6	4.2	−1.7	10.5
Prostate	WM	19.0	21.0	1.2	8.7
Bladder	WM	7.1	7.5	0.6	5.6
	WF	2.1	2.0	−1.4	−4.8
Kidney	WM	4.3	4.5	0.6	4.7
	WF	2.0	2.1	0.7	5.0
Leukaemia	WM	9.4	9.2	−0.4	−2.1
	WF	5.7	5.2	−1.7	−8.8

For age adjustment the 1970 United States population was used as standard.
* WM, white male; WF, white female.

is substantial and comparable with that for the preceding 35 years, 1935 to 1970 (7 per cent). The overall increase in incidence rates is even more marked than mortality rates in the past decade, involving a wide range of organs besides the lung (table A.4).[6] Moreover, the increase in incidence for all sites is comparable with that when lung cancer is excluded (table A.5).[7,8]

Table A.3 Crude cancer mortality rates per 100,000 population for selected sites by sex and year, England and Wales, 1971-77, and average per cent change[6]

Site	Sex	Mortality rate per 100,000		Average % change 1971-77	
		1971	1977	Annual	6-Year
All sites	M	265	283	1.1	6.8
	F	215	233	1.3	8.4
Stomach	M	30	28	−1.2	−6.7
	F	21	19	−1.7	−9.5
Large intestine	M	30	32	1.1	6.7
and rectum	F	34	35	0.4	2.9
Respiratory	M	106	112	0.9	5.7
	F	22	29	5.3	31.8
Breast	F	45	47	0.7	4.4
Uterus	F	15	16	1.1	6.7
Prostate	M	17	19	1.9	11.8
Bladder	M	12	12	0.0	0.0
	F	4.1	5.1	3.7	4.4
Leukaemia	M	7.0	7.2	0.4	2.9
	F	5.5	6.0	1.5	9.1

Reliance on overall age-adjusted incidence or mortality rates alone is simplistic, as such rates can mask steep increases in organ-specific cancers in high risk population subgroups, such as asbestos insulation workers or menopausal women treated with oestrogen replacement therapy. The overall probability, at today's death rates, of a person born now getting cancer by the age of 85 is 27 per cent for both men and women; this is increased from the 19 per cent for men and 22 per cent for women born in 1950.[9] Furthermore, recent cancer rate trends reflect exposures and events beginning some 20 or 30 years ago, when the production of synthetic organic chemicals was relatively trivial compared with the present levels. The production of synthetic organic compounds in the United States in 1935, 1950 and 1975 was about 1, 30 and 300 billion pounds per annum, respectively;[10] sharp increases have also been observed for a wide range of derived industrial products such as chlorinated hydrocarbon solvents, plastics and resin materials, and of industrial carcinogens, such as vinyl chloride and acrylonitrile. It is reasonable to anticipate that greater production has been paralleled by increased exposure of increasing numbers of both the workforce and the general public, which is likely further to accentuate increasing trends in cancer rates. It must also be recognised that before the 1976 Toxic Substances

Table A.4 Age-adjusted cancer incidence rates per 100,00 US population (whites) for selected sites by sex and year, 1969–76, and average per cent change[4]

Site	Sex	Incidence rate per 100,000		Average % change, 1969–76	
		1969	1976	Annual	7-Year
All sites	M	346.6	374.0	1.3	7.9
	F	271.5	301.2	2.0	10.9
Stomach	M	15.4	12.6	−2.3	−18.2
	F	7.1	5.6	−3.7	−21.1
Colon	M	34.5	36.9	1.5	7.0
	F	30.6	31.4	0.7	2.6
Rectum	M	17.5	19.4	1.3	10.9
	F	11.1	11.4	1.2	2.7
Pancreas	M	12.1	11.5	−0.5	−5.0
	F	7.5	8.0	0.9	6.7
Lung	M	70.6	77.8	1.4	10.2
	F	13.3	23.7	8.6	78.2
Melanoma	M	4.4	6.8	6.8	54.5
	F	4.1	6.1	6.2	48.8
Breast	F	73.9	83.5	1.8	13.0
Cervix	F	16.0	10.6	−5.9	−33.8
Uterus	F	22.6	31.2	5.9	38.1
Ovary	F	14.9	13.6	−0.4	8.7
Prostate	M	59.0	68.6	2.3	16.3
Bladder	M	23.8	26.4	2.3	10.9
	F	6.3	7.3	2.5	15.9
Kidney	M	9.0	9.6	1.2	6.7
	F	4.3	4.8	1.3	11.6
Leukaemia	M	13.2	13.1	−0.2	−0.8
	F	8.0	7.1	−1.0	−11.3

The 1970 population was used as standard for age-adjustment.

Act, which the chemical industry so effectively stalled for so long,[11] there were no requirements for testing chemicals before their introduction into commerce (with the exception of special-purpose legislation for drugs, pesticides and food additives). Thus, the overwhelming majority of industrial chemicals now in use have never been tested for chronic toxic and carcinogenic effects, let alone for ecological effects.

Role of smoking

As emphasised in *The Politics of Cancer*[1] (p. 178), 'Smoking is the single

Table A.5 Changes in US cancer incidence rates from 1970 to 1975[7,8]

	Average % increase in incidence rates, 1970–75			
	Cancers of all sites		Cancers of all sites except lung	
Groups	Annual	5-Year	Annual	5-Year
White male	0.9	4.7	0.9	4.6
Non-white male	2.3	11.9	2.7	14.3
White female	2.2	11.6	1.8	10.2
Non-white female	6.1	34.6	5.7	32.2

most important cause of lung cancer, as well as of cancer at other sites, chronic bronchitis and emphysema, and cardiovascular diseases'. Less well appreciated by lifestyle advocates is that overemphasis on smoking is widely used to divert attention from occupational causes of lung and other cancers. Of the approximately 100,000 annual lung cancer deaths in the United States, at least 20 per cent occur in nonsmokers. It is relevant that lung cancer death rates in nonsmokers approximately doubled[12] from 1958 to 1969, an increase maintained since. Furthermore, the role of occupational exposure to carcinogens was not recognised in most of the classic epidemiological studies which linked lung cancer with smoking. This led to overestimation of the contribution of smoking compared with occupational risks or to their possible interactions.

Thus, 'we are unable to say how much of the risks attributed to cigarettes is a "pure" cigarette risk and how much is cigarette times another, possibly on the job hazard'.[8] Moreover, smoking and occupation are confounded variables, smoking among men being more prevalent in 'blue-collar' workers than in professional and managerial classes.[13] Occupational causes of lung cancer include asbestos, radon daughters, nickel ores, chromium, arsenic, beryllium, mustard gas, vinyl chloride and bischloromethyl ether, apart from incompletely identified carcinogens in a wide range of industries such as rubber curing, tanning, steel (coke ovens), foundries, automobile, and petro-chemicals. Thus, lung cancer rates in asbestos insulation and topside coke oven workers are as much as 10 times greater than general population rates.

Underestimation of the role of such occupational carcinogens has been assisted by the fact that lung cancer mortality rates, based on the International Classification of Diseases, fail to distinguish pleural mesotheliomas from lung cancers; there is evidence of under-reporting of mesotheliomas (by about 75%) in high risk groups,[14] and even more so in occupations, such as automobile mechanics, where asbestos exposure has not been well recognised. There is a further lack of distinction between lung cancers of different histological types, some of which, such as adenocarcinomas, are less likely to be due to smoking than to occupational carcinogens.[15,16] 'In several instances where the risk of bronchogenic carcinoma has been shown to be increased among occupationally exposed groups, there has been an accompanying shift in the distribution of histologic types of tumours', away from the small-cell undifferentiated and squamous cell carcinoma of the lung, the principal types whose frequency is increased by smoking, in the direction of other types, particularly adenocarcinoma.[16] 'This (shift) has been noted among metal miners, uranium miners, copper smelter workers, vinyl chloride poly-merisation workers, chloromethyl methyl ether production workers, and mustard gas manufacturers'.[16]

Possible variations of smoking patterns fail to account for the marked excess in US lung cancer rates identified in specific occupational exposures, particularly among ethnic minorities and migrants from southern states.[17] A further challenge to the dominant role ascribed to smoking seems to be provided by observations that the risk of lung cancer in certain occupational groups, such as American Indian uranium miners,[18] Swedish zinc-lead miners,[19] mustard gas workers,[20] copper smelters exposed to arsenic,[21] and chloromethy methyl ether workers,[22] is about as high among nonsmokers as smokers, although the latency period is reduced in smokers, suggesting a possible promotional effect of smoking. It appears that the relative risks of lung cancer for smokers as against risks for nonsmokers may have been overestimated, particularly in less than lifetime studies.[23] Variations in smoking do not account for geographic excesses in lung cancer rates in US males and females, which overall reflect proximity of residence to petrochemical and certain other industries;[23,24] there are also data showing associations between levels of atmospheric carcinogens and lung cancer mortality rates.[25] It may be noted that a report[26] from Peto's own institution demonstrates that the correlation coefficient between lung cancer and smoking internationally explains only one-third as much of the variation as does the correlation between lung cancer and solid fuel consumption (0.4 versus 0.7; $r^2 = 0.16$ versus 0.49).

Overemphasis on the carcinogenic effects of smoking, and ignoring or discounting the role of occupational and other exposures, is extended by Peto and others to cancers of the bladder and pancreas which are variously characterised as related to or caused by smoking.[27,28] However, the relative risks for these cancers are several times less in smokers compared with nonsmokers than is the case for lung cancer. Excess bladder cancer rates have been identified in several occupational categories, including rubber, paint manufacturing and textile dyeing workers,[29] and among residents in highly industrialised countries,[30] particularly those with large chemical industry complexes.[31] Excess pancreatic cancer rates have also been reported in various occupations including steel and metal workers[32] and organic chemists.

Recognition of the important role of occupational exposures in lung cancers previously ascribed, exclusively or largely, to smoking in no way detracts from the recognition, emphasised in *The Politics of Cancer*, that the impact of smoking constitutes a 'national disaster'. There is no basis for regarding the smoking/lifestyle and occupational theories as mutually exclusive, particularly as these exposures may operate interactively. Furthermore, lifestyle is a somewhat misleading rubic for smoking as it restrictively implies voluntary personal choice. Placing responsibility for personal choice of an addictive lethal habit on young teenagers, the fastest growing group of new smokers, seems inappropriate. Failure to control smoking reflects a wide range of political and economic constraints, including massive press advertising by the industry which omits the word 'death' from the guarded small print warning of danger, massive revenues to federal, state and local government from tobacco taxes, federal subsidies to the industry and unwillingness of governments to increase tobacco taxation or to develop incentives to tobacco farmers to diversify. It is also important that the industry has moved to open up massive new markets with high-tar cigarettes in less developed countries, where the population is poorly informed on the hazards of smoking.

Role of diet

Lifestyle proponents are on less sure ground when they bracket diet, excess fat and overnutrition with smoking as the causes of the majority of cancer deaths. This claim is based largely on international correlations between consumption of total fat and rates for cancer of the breast and colon;[26] however, such correlations by themselves are not proof of causality. Similar correlations were found, in the same study from Peto's institution, between breast and colon cancers and other variables, such as Gross National Product and consumption of animal protein, which also appear to reflect industrialisation[26] (table A.6). Furthermore, 'epidemiologically, the case against fat is weak because there are populations that have a high fat intake and little bowel cancer . . .'.[33] Of two case control studies on the association between diet and breast cancer, one found no effect[34] and the other found trivial effects of fat and caloric intake, concluding that '. . . recommendations of major dietary modification as a possible preventive measure for breast cancer are clearly premature'.[35]

Table A.6 International correlations between breast, colon and liver cancers and possible aetiological variables[26]

	Correlation coefficients			
	Consumption of fat	Consumption of animal protein	Gross National Product	Total energy production
Breast cancer				
incidence	0.79	0.77	0.83	0.70
mortality	0.89	0.83	0.72	0.60
Colon cancer (M)				
incidence	0.74	0.74	0.81	0.68
mortality	0.85	0.86	0.77	0.69
Colon cancer (F)				
incidence	0.78	0.80	0.82	0.67
mortality	0.81	0.84	0.69	0.62
Liver cancer (M)				
incidence	−0.49	−0.59	−0.42	−0.25*
Liver cancer (F)				
incidence	−0.59	−0.67	−0.53	−0.31*

* Liquid energy.

Equally unconvincing are the studies, cited by Peto as corroborative evidence on the experimental effects of diet, which were largely concerned with the influence of fat on the incidence of tumours induced by chemical carcinogens and ionising radiation, and the influence of caloric intake on the incidence of spontaneous and induced tumours. Not only were different variables defined in the animal and human studies – per cent fat in the diet and total dietary fat, respectively – but increasing fat levels in the animal experiments were associated with increased incidence of skin, liver and breast cancers, whereas the reported correlations between fat consumption and liver cancer mortality are negative for both men and women (table A.6). Moreover, these experiments often failed to differentiate between variations of total dietary fat and caloric intake in test animals and to adjust caloric intake in controls to reflect dietary fat variations in test animals; the magnitude of the variations in fat and caloric intake required substantially to influence the incidence of induced and spontaneous tumours in experimental animals is generally far in excess of the dietary differences observed among the various human populations studied.[33] These experiments invariably failed to adjust the intake in controls of fat soluble carcinogens, present in fat as accidental environmental contaminants, to reflect variations of fat intake of test animals.

Peto's claim for the causal role of dietary fat in human cancer overstates the conclusions of those cited as the basis for his claims. Armstrong and Doll,[26] for instance, merely suggest that dietary fat levels may influence the incidence of colon and breast cancers, without asserting causality. Doll considers that diet may act by modifying the incidence of tumours induced by carcinogens or by acting as a vehicle for exogenous carcinogens[36] – a suggestion also made in *The Politics of Cancer* which Peto dismisses as 'implausible'. Carrol concludes that 'although caloric intake may be a factor in human carcinogenesis, it does not appear to offer a practical approach to the problem'.[37] As recognised by current concepts on the multifactorial aetiology of cancer, there is a substantial probability that a wide range of influences, diet and other lifestyle factors included, modify individual responses to carcinogenic agents. To ascribe causality to any particular modifying factor requires a degree of scientific evidence that has not yet been presented for dietary fat.

Role of occupation

Peto associates himself with the insistence by the chemical industry[2] and other lifestyle proponents that occupational exposures account for about 5 per cent[38,39,40] or 'a very small proportion'[41] of all cancers. This view is based on ascribing given percentages to known or alleged lifestyle factors, including smoking, fatty diet and sunlight, leaving a small unaccounted-for residue to which occupational factors are arbitrarily assigned by exclusion. The authors of this simplistic hypothesis compensate for its tenuous basis by reliance on 'educated estimates' and by making circular references to each other, often by 'personal communication', as the responsible authority.

However, there are problems with such 'guesstimates'. First, they fail to consider the multifactorial aetiology of cancer and the role of multiple causal agents, such as asbestos and smoking;[42] thus, the summation of known causes of cancer should properly exceed 100 per cent. As one of the lifestyle authors recently stressed,[36] 'there is now strong evidence to suggest that the risk of cancer is commonly increased by interaction of two or more factors'. Second, current cancer rates reflect exposures 20 to 30 years ago, when production levels of occupational carcinogens were a small fraction of the present; such estimates should thus now be adjusted to reflect increasing numbers of workers exposed. Third, the authors of these guesstimates failed to consider the very limited nature of the data on exposure to occupational carcinogens. Nor have they at any stage protested or even commented on the persistent refusal of the chemical industry to make such critical data available. In the absence of exposure data, it is even less clear how the 'lifestylers' confidently arrive at their estimate of less than 5 per cent.

Rather than addressing himself to such problems, Peto dismisses recent estimates of the importance of occupational carcinogens in a report by the US Public Health Service[43] as exaggerated, unsound and unreasonable. This report, prepared by nine named and internationally recognised experts in cancer epidemiology, statistics and carcinogenesis from three federal research agencies, is based on a National Occupational Hazard Survey which between 1972 and 1974 surveyed nearly 5,000 workplaces chosen to provide a cross-section of industry in the United States. The report estimated the total number of workers exposed to asbestos, nickel ores, chromium, arsenic, benzene and petroleum fractions, including aromatics. The excess cancers attributable to each of these carcinogens were derived by multiplying the number of exposed workers by known risk ratios and subtracting the 'normal incidence' of the cancer.

The report concluded that 'as much as 20% or more' of cancers in the near term and future may reflect past exposure to the six carcinogens considered. The uncertainties and limitations in these conclusions, including the possibility that exposures and risk ratios may have been overestimated in some instances, were clearly stated in the report, as were other considerations including the multifactorial aetiology of cancer, and the role of lifestyle factors and their possible interactions with occupational exposures.

The possibility that this government report underestimates rather than overestimates the role of occupational exposures, for several reasons some of which are recognised in the report, has not been considered by its denigrators, including Peto. First, the calculations in the report ignore the role of radiation and of some ten epidemiologically recognised occupational carcinogens, other than the six considered. Second, the risk ratios considered may be artificially low as they were largely derived from less-than-lifetime epidemiological studies, which may thus underestimate the true risk in view of the long latencies commonly involved. Third, the report does not consider the many statistical and methodological constraints common to most occupational epidemiological studies[44] such as relatively small numbers of workers in many locations, changes in exposure patterns over time due to employee turnover, plant shutdown, process and production changes and changes in management, all of which lead to fragmentation of health and exposure records, access to which is often restricted by industry. Fourth, the estimates fail to take account of the many chemicals recognised as carcinogenic in animals for which there are no exposure or epidemiological data. Thus, of 442 chemicals and industrial processes recently evaluated by the International Agency for

Research on Cancer (IARC), epidemiological data are available for only 60 (14 per cent), although evidence of experimental carcinogenicity was considered to be sufficient for 143 (32 per cent).[45] Fifth, the estimates exclude high risk occupations with incompletely defined carcinogens, such as the steel, rubber and tanning industries. Sixth, the estimates do not adequately reflect conditions in small business where exposure levels are likely to be higher than in major chemical companies. Seventh, the report does not reflect major increases in the production of the occupational carcinogens it considered such as benzene, with the likelihood of recently increasing exposures. Eighth, the study examined only a limited number of sites, excluding cancers such as skin and bladder which are known to be occupationally related. Finally, the estimates neglect the possible role of fugitive point-source emissions of industrial carcinogens as causes for the excess of overall and organ-specific cancers, including lung, bladder, colon, pancreas and breast, in residents of certain highly industrialised counties.

This government report has received extensive support from various expert bodies, such as the Toxic Substances Strategy Committee, whose position has been endorsed by 17 federal agencies, and international groups, such as the International Labour Organisation, and the US and British trades unions. The report has also received additional support in the critique of two consultants to the chemical industry's American Industrial Health Council which concluded that '. . . the full range [of total cancer attributable to occupational exposure] using multiple classifications may be from 10 to 33 per cent or perhaps higher if we had better information on some other potentially carcinogenic substances . . . The annual number of cancer deaths attributable to asbestos is in the range from 29,700 to 54,000, which corresponds to a percentage range of the total cancer of 7 to 14 per cent . . . Any argument over these numbers cannot detract from the fact that asbestos exposure was, as the authors [of the Government report] state, a major public health disaster . . . We also believe that reduction of exposure to carcinogens in the course of employment can certainly be expected to effect major reductions in the frequencies of occurrence of cancer and is one of the most promising applications of preventive medicine'.[47] The American Industrial Health Council failed to release this critique until the record of the recent Occupational Safety and Health Administration hearings on regulation of occupational carcinogens closed.

Conclusions

Cancer is a disease of multifactorial aetiology to which occupational exposure and smoking can contribute importantly, sometimes interactively. There have been substantial recent increases in cancer rates which cannot be accounted for by smoking alone. Smoking is the major lifestyle factor of importance in cancer, and evidence for the causal role of other lifestyle factors, particularly diet, is slender. The role of lifestyle factors has been exaggerated, by those with an economic or intellectual investment in this theory, by largely excluding involuntary exposures to carcinogens and minimising the role of occupational carcinogens. These considerations further illustrate the primary thesis of *The Politics of Cancer*: cancer is essentially a preventable disease which requires intervention and regulation at several levels, particularly the occupational and smoking. Failure to prevent cancer reflects major political and economic constraints which have hitherto been largely unrecognised or discounted.

Notes

1. Peto, R. *Nature* **284**, 297–300 (1980).
2. Epstein, S. S. *The Politics of Cancer* (Sierra Club Books, San Francisco, 1978, revised and expanded in Anchor/Doubleday, New York, 1979); quotations refer to the 1979 edition.
3. *AIHC Recommended Alternatives to OSHA's Generic Carcinogen Proposal, Occupational Safety & Health Administration (OSHA) Docket No. H-090)* (American Industrial Health Council, 24 February, 1978).
4. *Vital Statistics—Special Reports, U.S. DHEW*, **43**, 163 (1956); *Vital Statistics of the U.S.* **2** (1970).
5. Pollack, E. S. & Horm, J. W. *J. natn. Cancer Inst.* **64**, 1091 (1980).
6. *Trends in Mortality, 1951–1975* (U.K. Office of Population Censuses and Surveys, Series DH1, No. 3, 1978).
7. *Third National Cancer Survey, 1969–1971 (NCI, Bethesda)*; *Cancer Surveillance Epidemiology and End Results (SEER) Program*.
8. Schneiderman, M. *Occupational Safety & Health Administration OSHA Docket 090* (4 April, 1978).
9. Zdeb, M. S. *Am. J. Epidemiol.* **106**, 6 (1977).
10. Davis, D. L. & Magee, B. H. *Science* **206**, 1356 (1979); see also U.S. International Trade Commission Reports.
11. *Chemical Dangers in the Workplace*, 34th Report of the

Committee on Government Operations, House of Representatives (September 27, 1976).

12. Enstrom, J. E. *J. natn. Cancer Inst.* **62**, 755 (1979).

13. Sterling, T. D. *Int. J. Hlth Services* **8**, 437 (1978).

14. Newhouse, M. L. & Wagner, J. C. *Br. J. ind. Med.* **26**, 302 (1969).

15. Wynder, E. L. & Stellman, S. D. *Cancer Res.* **37**, 4608 (1977).

16. Wagoner, J. K., Infante, P. F. & Bayliss, D. L. *Envir. Res.* **21**, 15 (1980).

17. Mancuso, T. F. & Sterling, T. D. *J. natn. med. Ass.* **67**, 107 (1975).

18. Archer, V. E., Gilliam, J. D. & Wagoner, J. K. *Ann. N.Y. Acad. Sci.* **271**, 280 (1976).

19. Axelson, O. & Sundell, L. *Scand. J. Work envir. Hlth* **4**, 46 (1978).

20. Yamada, A. *Acta path. jap.* **13**, 131 (1963).

21. Pinto, S. S. *Archs envir. Hlth* **33**, 325 (1978).

22. Weiss, W. & Boucot, K. R. *J. Am. med. Ass.* **234**, 1139 (1975).

23. Mason, J. T. & McKay, F. W. *Atlas of Cancer Mortality for U.S. Counties: 1950–1969* (Dept H.E.W., Washington, D.C., 1975); *Atlas of Cancer Mortality for U.S. Counties among U.S. Non-Whites* (Dept H.E.W., Washington, D.C., 1976).

24. Blot, W. J. *et al. Science* **198**, 51 (1977).

25. Carnow, B. *Envir. Hlth Perspect.* **22**, 17 (1978).

26. Armstrong, B. K. & Doll, R. *Int. J. Cancer* **15**, 617 (1975).

27. Cole, P., Monson, R. R., Haning, H. & Friedell, G. H. *New Engl. J. Med.* **284**, 129 (1971).

28. Wynder, E. L., Mabuchi, K., Maruch, N. & Fortner, J. G. *Cancer* **31**, 641 (1973).

29. Cole, P. & Goldman, R. *Persons at High Risk of Cancer: An Approach to Cancer Etiology and Control* (ed. Fraumeni, J. F. Jr) 167–184 (Academic, New York, 1975).

30. Blot. W. J. & Fraumeni, J. *J. natn. Cancer Inst.* **61**, 1017 (1978).

31. Hoover, R. & Fraumeni, J. *Envir. Res.* **9**, 196 (1975).

32. Milham, J. in *Occupational Carcinogenesis* (eds Wagoner, J. & Saffiotti, U.) 243–249 (New York Academy of Sciences, 1976).

33. Berg. J. W. in *Persons at High Risk of Cancer: An Approach to Cancer Etiology and Control* (ed. Fraumeni, J. F. Jr) 210–224 (Academic, New York, 1975).

34. Phillips, R. L. *Cancer Res.* **35**, 3513 (1975).

35. Miller, A. B. *et al. Am. J. Epidemiol.* **107**, 499 (1978).

36. Doll, R. *Cancer Res.* **45**, 2475 (1980).

37. Caroll, K. K. *Cancer Res.* **35**, 3374 (1975).

38. Higginson, J. & Muir, C. S. *J. natn. Cancer Inst.* **63**, 1291 (1979).

39. Wynder, E. L. & Gori, G. B. *Am. J. Publ. Hlth* **66**, 359 (1977).

40. Maugh, T. H. *Science* **205**, 1363 (1979).

41. Doll, R. *Nature* **265**, 589 (1977).

42. Selikoff, I. J. & Hammond, C. E. *J. Am. med. Ass.* **242**, 458 (1979).

43. Bridbord, K. *et al. Estimates of the Fraction of Cancer in the United States Related to Occupational Factors* (National Cancer Institute, National Institute of Environmental Health Sciences, and National Institute for Occupational Safety and Health, 15 September, 1978).

44. Stellman, J. M. & Stellman, S. D. *What Proportion of Cancer is Attributable to Occupation; Statistical and Social Consideration* (American Society for Preventive Oncology, Chicago, 6–7 March, 1980).

45. Report of an IARC Working Group *Cancer Res.* **40**, 1 (1980).

46. *Toxic Chemicals and Public Protection* (Report to the President of the Toxic Substances Strategy Committee of the Council on Environmental Quality, May, 1980).

47. Stallones, R. A. & Downs, T. *A Critical Review of Bridbord, K. et al.* prepared for the American Industrial Health Council (1979).

Theories of Cancer*

Sir – In reviewing my book *The Politics of Cancer*,[1] Peto[2] charged that one table (Table 6.4) selectively and deliberately omitted data that would otherwise have questioned the conclusion that low dietary doses of saccharin (0.01 per cent) are carcinogenic in rats. This statement is incorrectly based on comparison of Table 6.4 with data in an appendix to the report of the Office of Technology Assessment.[3] However, the caption of Table 6.4 clearly states that it is based on another table, prepared by Melvin Reuber for use in the congressional testimony on saccharin by the Health Research Group on 21 March 1977.[4] Peto persisted in publishing this serious allegation in spite of two warnings.

Peto also appears unfamiliar with the content of the Office of Technology Assessment's report, which he cites as the basis for his charges on saccharin. This report explicitly discusses Reuber's low-dose data and his conclusion that 'the increased incidence of lymphosarcoma of the thorax

---

*Letter from Samuel Epstein to the editor of *Nature* (vol. 289, 15 January 1981) in response to Richard Peto's article (reprinted as appendix 2, this book).

in rats at the 0.01 per cent . . . are highly significant in the saccharin study'.[5] Reuber also emphasises that the carcinogenic effects of saccharin in various studies were not always dose-related.

Contrary to Peto's impressions, inversions in dose-response data are not uncommon in both experimental and epidemiological carcinogenicity studies. Reasons for such inversions include competing risks, heterogeneity in tested populations, and statistical fluctuation, particularly when dose-response curves are shallow. Peto also fails to recognise that saccharin has produced tumours in experimental animals at low as well as at relatively high doses.

Contrary to Peto's impression that 'it is not surprising that so many chemicals (such as saccharin) at such (high) doses can cause cancer in animals,' there is an overwhelming consensus in the qualified, independent scientific community that high-dose testing does not produce false positive results, and that this is necessary to reduce the insensitivity of carcinogenicity tests, reflecting the small number of animals tested compared with large human populations at presumptive risk.[6] It is also well recognised that carcinogenicity testing in excess of maximally tolerated doses (MTD) can produce false negatives due to competing toxicity.

Peto's charge of selective omission of the saccharin data is not his only misrepresentation. After his circulation of drafts of his review to various US experts in the autumn of 1979, Schneiderman, then Associate Director for Science Policy of the National Cancer Institute (NCI) and co-author of the government report on the importance of occupational carcinogens,[7] explained in a letter to Peto that breast cancer correlates as well with Gross National Product as fat, that occupation had been ignored in studies exclusively associating lung cancer with smoking, that there have been major recent increases in lung cancer among non-smokers and that there have been 'big and frightening' recent increases in cancer incidence which cannot be accounted for by smoking or other lifestyle factors.

Similarly, Upton, then Director of NCI and a co-author of the report,[7] challenged the erroneous charge that a '4–5' multiplication factor was used to inflate the 1978 government estimates of cancer anticipated from occupational exposures. '. . . This simply is not true . . .'

Repeatedly, Peto dismisses as personal views statements in *The Politics of Cancer* to which he takes exception, rather than recognising that they are based on fully referenced primary sources and without attempting to challenge these sources directly. For instance, he disparages the conclusion 'that the cure rates for major cancers have not been improving much over recent years' without noting that this reflects cited NCI data. Peto refers to the 'claims that cancer costs the US economy over $25 billion per year' without recognising that such figures are derived from NCI sources. Similarly, Peto criticises as 'misleading or unbalanced' references to the term 'medical-industrial complex' without attribution to its source, referenced and identified in the text (p. 77), as the caption of an editorial in *The Lancet*.[8]

Peto charges that the book denigrates the value of short-term carcinogenicity tests, which he asserts is a 'most inexplicable error of scientific judgement.' While problems of such tests, particularly the limited associations between carcinogenicity and Ames test data for compounds from a wide range of structural classes[9,10] are recognised, the book concludes (p. 68) that there is a 'range of useful applications' for these tests, particularly when incorporated into battery protocols.

Peto accepts that industries 'delay or obstruct any hygienic measures which will cost money. . . . (and) that the scientific literature is not immune from distortion by financial interests.'[11] Peto apparently also accepts the wide range of case studies in *The Politics of Cancer*, which document a common pattern of constraints, including manipulation, distortion and destruction, in health, safety and economic data generated or interpreted by industry and its consultants. Yet he seems willing to accept studies sponsored or endorsed by industry as authority for the nearly exclusive lifestyle theory of cancer causation. Moreover, he is opposed to further regulatory controls on grounds of costs, professed 'inactive conservatism', and because 'for most toxic chemicals, we now have both qualitative and quantitative uncertainty about the health benefits of restriction.' This seems a questionable basis for prudent public health policy.

Samuel S. Epstein
*School of Public Health,
University of Illinois at the
Medical Center, Chicago, Illinois*

1. Epstein, S. S. *The Politics of Cancer* (Sierra Club Books, San Francisco 1978, revised and expanded in Anchor/Doubleday, New York, 1979, to which quotations refer).

2. Peto. R. *Nature* **284**, 297–300 (1980).

3. *Cancer Testing Technology and Saccharin* U.S. Congress, Washington, D.C., June 7, 1977.

4. Wolfe, S. M. Johnson, A. *Public Citizens Health Research Group, Testimony Before Subcommittee on Health, House Commerce Committee Hearings on Saccharin*, March 21, 1977.

5. Reuber, M. D. *Envir. Hlth Perspect.* **25**, 173 (1978).

6. Report to the Surgeon General, USPHS, *Evaluation of*

Environmental Carcinogens (*Ad Hoc* Committee on the Evaluation of Low Levels of Environmental Chemical Carcinogens, April 22, 1970).

7. Bridbord, K. *et al. Estimates of the Fraction of Cancer in the United States Related to Occupational Factors* (NCI, National Institute of Environmental Health Sciences, and National Institute for Occupational Safety and Health, 15 September, 1978).

8. *Lancet* **ii**, 1380 (1973).

9. Rinkus, S. J. & Legator, M. S. *Cancer Res.* **39** 3289 (1979).

10. *International Program for the Evaluation of Short Term Tests for Carcinogenicity* National Toxicology Program. Dept of Health and Human Services, April, 1980).

Appendix 4. Relevant prescribed diseases*

Description of disease	Nature of occupation
Squamous-celled carcinoma of the skin.	Any occupation involving: The use or handling of, or exposure to, arsenic, tar, pitch, bitumen, mineral oil (including paraffin), soot or any compound, product (including quinone or hydroquinone), or residue of any of these substances.
Malignant diseases of the skin or subcutaneous tissues or of the bones, or due to electro-magnetic radiations (other than radiant heat), or to ionising particles.	Exposure to electro-magnetic radiations other than radiant heat, or to ionising particles.
Carcinoma of the mucous membrane of the nose or associated air sinuses. Primary carcinoma of a bronchus or of a lung.	Work in a factory where nickel is produced by decomposition of a gaseous nickel compound which necessitates working in or about a building or buildings where that process or any other industrial process ancillary or incidental thereto is carried on.

Primary neoplasm of the epithelial lining of the urinary bladder (Papilloma of the bladder), or of the renal pelvis or of the ureter or of the urethra.	(a) Work in a building in which any of the following substances is produced for commercial purposes:
	  (i) Alpha-naphthylamine or beta-naphthylamine;
	  (ii) Diphenyl substituted by at least one nitro or primary amino group or by at least one nitro and primary amino group;
	  (iii) Any of the substances mentioned in sub-paragraph (ii) above if further ring substituted by halogeno, methyl or methoxy groups, but not by other groups;

* Information in this appendix taken from Leaflet NI 2, *Prescribed Industrial Diseases*, DHSS.

Description of disease	Nature of occupation
	(iv) The salts of any of the substances mentioned in sub-paragraphs (i) to (iii) above;
	(v) Auramine or magenta;
	(b) The use or handling of any of the substances mentioned in sub-paragraphs (i) to (iv) of paragraph (a), or work in process in which any such substance is used or handled or is liberated;
	(c) the maintenance of any plant or machinery used in any such process as is mentioned in paragraph (b), or the cleaning of clothing used in any such building as is mentioned in paragraph (a) if such clothing is cleaned within the works of which the building forms a part or in a laundry maintained and used solely in connection with such works.
Primary malignant neoplasm of the mesothelium (diffuse mesothelioma) of the pleura or of the peritoneum.	(a) The working or handling of asbestos or any admixture of asbestos;
	(b) the manufacture or repair of asbestos textiles or other articles containing or composed of asbestos;
	(c) the cleaning of any machinery or plant used in any of the foregoing operations and of any chambers, fixtures and appliances for the collection of asbestos dust;
	(d) substantial exposure to the dust arising from any of the foregoing operations.
Adeno-carcinoma of the nasal cavity or associated air sinuses.	Attendance for work in or about a building where wooden furniture is manufactured.
Angiosarcoma of the liver.	Work in or about machinery or apparatus used for the polymerisation of vinyl chloride monomer, a process which, for the purposes of this provision, comprises all operations up to and including the drying of the slurry produced by the polymerisation and the packaging of the dried product; or work in a building or structure in which any part of the aforementioned process takes place.

Appendix 5. Sample agreement on carcinogens*

NGA members at the *East Anglian Daily Times* in Ipswich have been successful in reaching an agreement about the use of chemicals, and particularly those which are suspected of causing cancer.

The Agreement states that the *East Anglian Daily Times*

> shall endeavour to substitute any chemical of known or suspected carcinogenic potential with a safer product. If substitution is not possible, a mutually agreed safe working practice shall be drawn up aimed at eliminating risk.

In defining which chemicals are suspected of causing cancer, sources of information will include the Health and Safety Executive, the United States National Institute of Occupational Safety and Health, and the International Agency for Research on Cancer.

All chemicals used at the *East Anglian Daily Times* will be investigated before they are put into use. Preliminary trials may be in conjunction with atmospheric monitoring to ensure that agreed limits are not being threatened.

The Carcinogens Agreement has been made in conjunction with the drawing up of the East Anglian Daily Times Company Safety Policy. This management policy recognises the rights of safety representatives to be consulted about health and safety matters, to have proper facilities to do their job, to consult outside bodies or independent experts, to have access to the company health and safety library and to be involved in the formulation of safe working practices.

In addition, the safety policy entitles safety representatives to time off work without loss of pay to carry out any of their duties and to attend training and retraining provided by the TUC, their trade union and any other course approved by their trade union.

The policy also states that all data sheets shall be catalogued and copies kept in the First Aid Room, Production Office and Union Office. No

* This appendix is based on a press release, issued by the NGA (14 May 1982)

chemicals may be brought into use without first consulting the Safety Officer who will inform the Safety Representative. All containers must be clearly marked as to their content.

John Willats, NGA National Officer with responsibilities for health and safety comments:

> This agreement represents a considerable achievement on the part of the NGA Chapel at the *East Anglian Daily Times*. I hope that it will serve as an example to other union members.
>
> It shows that such agreements are possible and that they are an important part of our strategy to control the use of chemicals in the printing industry.
>
> It is the particular aim of the NGA to rid this industry of all known and suspected carcinogens, which we believe to be a significant threat to print workers.

Agreement between NGA Production Chapel and East Anglia Daily Times (EADT) Company regarding safety of chemistry used

These points of agreement should be read in conjunction with the EADT Health and Safety document and do not in any way reduce EADT's responsibility under the Health and Safety at Work Act.

Monitoring of possible health hazards

If a chemical in use, or proposed to be used, contains or is reasonably suspected of containing, a known hazardous ingredient, the safety officer in consultation with the relevant safety representative, shall effect an immediate investigation. This may require atmospheric monitoring using either an outside agency or the use of proprietary environmental monitoring of an appropriate nature using relevant equipment, by the safety officer and safety representative. Where tests show that safety limits are being threatened or exceeded immediate steps shall be taken aimed at bringing the situation back within mutually acceptable limits.

Carcinogenic substances

The company shall endeavour to substitute any chemical of known or suspected carcinogenic potential with a safer product. If substitution is not possible, a mutually agreed safe working practice shall be drawn up aimed at eliminating risk.

On a regular basis, suppliers of chemicals will be asked to state if any of their products, which we use, contain any of the chemicals of known or suspected carcinogenic potential. In this regard, the following sources of information may be amongst those used:

1 Health and Safety Executive, *Guidance Note 15*
2 International Agency for Research on Cancer (World Health Organisation), *Chemicals and Industrial Processes Associated with Cancer in Humans*
3 National Institute for Occupational Safety of Health, current intelligence and bulletins
4 Health and Safety Executive, *Packing and Labelling of Dangerous Substances Regulation 1978 and 1981*

Appendix 6. Further reading on cancer prevention

Regular journals

As yet, there is no single journal primarily dealing with the wider issues of cancer prevention. However, we list below those journals which some-times carry relevant articles.

Ecologist, c/o Edward Goldsmith, 73 Molesworth Street, Wadebridge, Cornwall, PL27 7DS.
Hazards Bulletin, c/o BSSRS, 9 Poland Street, London W1V 3D.
Health and Safety at Work, c/o Maclaren Publishers Ltd, David House, 69–77 High Street, Croydon, CS 1QH.
International Journal of Health Services, c/o Baywood Publishing Co., 43 Central Drive, Formingade, NY 11735, USA.
Medicine in Society, c/o Marxists in Medicine, 16 King Street, London WC2E 8HY.
Radical Science Journal, c/o BSSRS, 9 Poland Street, London W1V 3DG.
Science for People, c/o BSSRS, 9 Poland Street, London W1V 3DG.

In addition, of course, there is a wide range of medical journals, both general and specialist, which if necessary can be consulted in a medical school library.

Books and Pamphlets

Association of Scientific, Technical and Management Staffs (ASTMS), *The Prevention of Occupational Cancer* (1980). Available from ASTMS, 10 Jamestown Road, London.
Boston Women's Health Book Collective, *Our Bodies Ourselves*, British edition by Angela Phillips and Jill Rakusen, Harmondsworth, Penguin (1980). Contains a specific discussion of cancer as it relates to women.

Bull, D., *A Growing Problem; Pesticides and the Third World Poor*, Oxfam (1982).

City University Statistical Laboratory and GMWU, *Cancer and Work* (1983).

Cook, J., and C. Kaufman, *Portrait of a Poison: The 2,4,5-T Story*, Pluto Press (1982). The story of the dioxin campaign from a trade union perspective.

Dalton, A., *Asbestos Killer Dust*, BSSRS (1979).

Delbridge, R., and M. Smith (eds), *Consuming secrets: How Official Secrecy Affects Everyday Life in Britain*, Burnett (1982). Contains excellent chapters on the environment and product testing.

Doll, R., and R. Peto, *The Causes of Cancer*, Oxford University Press (1981). For a critique of this viewpoint see Appendix 3.

Doyal, L., with I. Pennell, *The Political Economy of Health*, Pluto Press (1979). A general introduction to the social causes of ill-health in both the developed and underdeveloped world.

Epstein, S. S., *The Politics of Cancer*, Anchor Press (1979).

Epstein, S. S., L. O. Brown and C. Pope, *Hazardous Waste in America*, Sierra Club Books (1982).

Frankel, M., *Chemical Risk*, Pluto Press (1982). A useful guide to how you can find out about the possible risks of any chemical you are exposed to.

Frankel, M., *The Social Audit Pollution Handbook*, Macmillan (1978).

General & Municipal Workers Union, *A Preliminary Cancer Prevention Campaign* (1980) available from GMBATU, Thorne House, Ruxley Ridge, Claygate, Esher, Surrey KT10 0TI.

Hay, A., *The Chemical Scythe: lessons of 2,4,5-T and Dioxin*, Plenum (1982).

Kinnersly, P., *The Hazards of Work: How to Fight Them*, Pluto Press (1973). A detailed discussion of workplace hazards including carcinogens. Now somewhat out of date but a new edition is expected soon.

Kushner, R., *Breast Cancer: A Personal History and Investigative Report*, New York, Harcourt Brace Jovanovitch (1975).

Moss, R. W., *The Cancer Syndrome*, New York, Grove Press (1982). An excellent exposé of the politics of cancer research.

New Scientist, *The Risk Equation*, IPC Publications (1977). Contains some useful discussions of the general problems of controlling occupational and environmental hazards.

National Graphical Association (NGA), *Occupational Cancer in the*

Printing Industry (1980). Available from NGA, 63–67 Bromham Road, Bedford M40 2AG.

National Union of Agricultural and Allied Workers (NUAAW), *Not One Minute Longer* (1980). Available from NUAAW, Headland House, 30 Grays Inn Road, London WC1X 8DS.

Saffiotti, U., and J. M. Wagoner, *Occupational Carcinogens*, New York Academy of Sciences, vol. 271 (1976).

le Serve, A., C. Vose, C. Wigley and D. Bennett, *Chemicals, Work and Cancer*, Nelson (1980). An invaluable guide to cancer for workers.

Tait, N., *Asbestos Kills*, Spaid (1977). Available from Spaid, 38 Draper Road, Enfield, Middlesex EN2 8W. A campaigning book exposing the dangers of asbestos.

Appendix 7. Useful organisations

BSSRS Work Hazards groups

Birmingham
Health and Safety Advice Centre,
164 Edmund St, Birmingham B3,
Phone 021 236 0801.

Brighton
Work Hazards Group
J. Colover, Broyle Mill Farm, The
Broyle, Ringmer, Sussex.

London
BSSRS, 9 Poland St, London W1.
Phone 01-437 2728.

Women and Work Hazards Group
9 Poland St, London W1.
Phone 01-437 2728.

Manchester
D. Russell, 140 Epping Walk,
Hulme.

NE Hazards Group
13 Railway St, Langley Park,
Durham.
Phone 0385 731889.

Sheffield
PO Box 148,
Sheffield S1 1SB.

West Yorkshire
43 Leylands Lane, Bradford 9.
Phone 0274 43298.

Local TU Safety and Health groups

**Birmingham Region Union Safety
& Health Campaign**
Eric Shakespeare, 160 Corisande
Road, Birmingham B29.
Phone 021 471 1236.

Derby Area Safety & Health
Mike McLoughlin, 12 Wenlock
Close, Mickleover, Derby
DE3 5NT.
Phone 0332 518216.

**Harlow Trades Council H&S
Group**
Danny Purton, 9 Willowfield,
Harlow, Essex.
Phone 0279 31656.

Hull Action on Safety & Health
3 Ferens Avenue, Cottingham
Road, Hull HU6 7SY.
Phone 0482 497468.

Isle of Wight Trade Union Safety Group
Bob Davies, 12 Winston Road, Newport, IOW.

North East Lancashire Action on Safety & Health
Bill Greenwood, 52 Helmshore Road, Halingdon, Lancashire.

Leicester Area Safety Action Movement
Dave Adams, 6 Martin Close, Whitwick, Near Coalville, Leicestershire.
Phone 0530 36777.

London North –
North London Health & Safety
146 Kentish Town Road, London NW1 9QG.
Phone 01-485 6672.

London –
East London Health & Safety Group
341 Commercial Road, London E1.
Phone 01-791 0741.

Milton Keynes Association for Safety & Health
Ian Anderson, 46 Blackdown, Fullers Slade, Milton Keynes.
Phone 0908 564466.

Nottingham –
Greater Nottingham Action on Safety & Health
118 Mansfield Road, Nottingham.
Phone 0602 582369.

Rotherham –
Workers in Safety & Health
WEA Chantry Buildings, Corporation Street, Rotherham.
Phone 0709 72121.

Rugby Industrial Safety Centre
Bill Lawrence (Chairman), 68 Main Street, Long Lawford, Rugby.

Scotland – Dunfermline
Dunfermline Area Safety & Health Group
Les Cowey, 14 Markfield Road, Dalgety Bay, Fife, Scotland.

Scotland West –
West of Scotland Health & Safety Group
Alison West, WEA, 212 Bath Street, Glasgow G2 4HW.
Phone 041 332 0176.

Sheffield Area Trade Union Safety Committee
Seb Schmoller, 312 Albert Road, Heeley, Sheffield 8.
Phone 0742 584559.

Walsall Action for Safety & Health
George Mason, Schoolhouse, Teddesley Street, Walsall, West Midlands.
Phone 0922 30073.

Other organisations and groups

Action on Smoking and Health (ASH)
27 Mortimer Street, London
W1N 7RJ (tel. 01 637 9843).

British Society for Social Responsibility in Science (BSSRS)
c/o 9 Poland Street, London
W1V 3DG (tel. 01 437 2728).

Cancer Prevention Society
c/o E. Rushworth, 102 Inverary
Drive, Bearsden, Glasgow
G61 2AT.

Cancer Information Association
Gloucester Green, Oxford
OE1 2EQ (tel. 0865 46654).

Freedom of Information Campaign
c/o Mrs M. V. Butler, The
Cottage, Weir Courtney,
Lingfield, Surrey.

Friends of the Earth (FOE)
c/o 9 Poland Street, London
W1V 3DG.

Marxists in Medicine
16 St. John Street, London
EC1M 4AY.

Politics of Health Group
c/o 9 Poland Street, London
W1V 3DG.

Socialist Environment and Resources Association (SERA)
c/o 9 Poland Street, London
W1V 3DG (tel. 01 439 3749).

Socialist Medical Association (SMA)
c/o 9 Poland Street, London
W1V 3DG (tel. 01 439 3395).

SPAID
c/o Nancy Tait, 38 Drapers Road,
Enfield, Middlesex EN2 8LU.

Women's National Cancer Control Campaign
9 King Street, London WC2E 8HN
(tel. 01 830 9901).

Appendix 8. Members of the Advisory Committee on Toxic Substances as of June 1982

D. J. Barnett (Association of District Councils Nominee), Chief Environmental Health Officer, Bristol City Council.

J. R. Boddy (TUC Nominee), General Secretary, National Union of Agricultural and Allied Workers.

T. A. Connors (HSE Nominee), Director, Medical Research Council, Toxicology Unit.

G. M. Davies (HSE Nominee), Occupational Hygiene Unit Research Centre, British Steel Corporation.

H. J. Dunster (Chairperson), Deputy-Director General, HSE.

J. F. Eccles (TUC Nominee), Regional Secretary, National Union of General and Municipal Workers.

N. G. Fiske (CBI Nominee), National Farmers Union.

J. P. Hamilton (TUC Nominee), Social Insurance and Industrial Welfare Department, TUC.

P. M. Heron (CBI Nominee), BP International.

C. Jenkins (TUC Nominee), General Secretary, Association of Scientific, Technical and Managerial Staffs.

I. G. Laing (CBI Nominee), Technical Director, Clayton Aniline Co Ltd.

S. H. Moore (Association of Metropolitan Authorities Nominee) Metropolitan Borough of Rochdale.

R. S. F. Schilling OBE (HSE Nominee).

M. Sharratt (HSE Nominee), Occupational Health Unit, Research Centre, BP Co Ltd.

K. S. Williamson (CBI Nominee), Principal Medical Officer, ICI.

Appendix 9. Members of the Food Additives and Contaminants Committee as of January 1982

B. C. L. Weedon (Chairperson), Vice-Chancellor, University of Nottingham.

R. B. Beedham, Production and Technical Director, Smedley-HP Foods Ltd.

P. J. Brignell, Manager of the Corporate Intelligence Unit at Imperial Chemical Industries Ltd.

J. R. Cockcroft, Chairperson of the Consumers' Committee for England and Wales and Great Britain; Chairperson of the United Nations' Status of Women Commission.

J. W. Colquhoun, Director of Products Research and Development Group, Rowntree Mackintosh.

W. Elstow, Director of Joint General Manager of Weston Research Laboratories Ltd.

T. T. Gorsuch, Director of Research, Reckitt and Colman Ltd.

A. J. Harrison, Chief Scientific Adviser, Public Analyst and Agricultural Analyst, Avon and Gloucestershire County Councils.

I. Macdonald, Professor of Applied Physiology, Guy's Hospital Medical School.

D. S. McLaren, Reader, Department of Physiology, University of Edinburgh.

J. W. G. Porter, Director of National Institute for Research in Dairying, University of Reading.

P. P. Scott, Professor of Nutrition and Physiology, Royal Free Hospital Medical School, University of London.

P. Turner, Professor of Clinical Pharmacology, St Bartholomew's Hospital; Chairperson of the Committee on Toxicity of Chemicals in Food, Consumer Products and the Environment.

Appendix 10. Independent members of the Advisory Committee on Pesticides and its scientific subcommittee as of December 1980

The Advisory Committee on Pesticides

R. Kilpatrick, CBE, MD, FRCPEd, FRCP (Chairperson), Dean of the School of Medicine, University of Leicester.

R. L. Carter, MA, DM, DSc, FRCPath, Reader in Pathology, Institute of Cancer Research, Consultant Pathologist, Royal Marsden Hospital, Hon. Consultant Pathologist, MRC Toxicology Unit, Carshalton.

L. E. Coles, BPharm, PhD, CChem, MPhA, MChemA, FPS, FRSC, County Analyst and Agricultural Analyst, Mid-Glamorgan Public Health Laboratory, Cardiff.

R. Goulding, BSc, MD, FRCP, FRCPath, Emeritus Consultant in Clinical Toxicology, Guys Hospital, London.

E. B. G. Jones, MSc, PhD, DSc, Professor and Director of Research, Department of Biological Sciences, Portsmouth Polytechnic.

J. Knowelden, MD, FRCP, FFCM, DPH, JP, Professor of Community Medicine, University of Sheffield.

R. I. McCallum, MD, DSc, FRCP, FFOM, Reader in Industrial Health and Head of Department of Occupational Health and Hygiene, University of Newcastle-upon-Tyne.

G. R. Sagar, MA, DPhil, Professor of Agricultural Botany, School of Plant Biology, University College of North Wales, Bangor.

R. S. Tayler, BSc (Agric), Dip Agric NDA, Senior Lecturer in Crop Production, University of Reading.

M. J. Way, MA, DSc, Director of Imperial College, Silwood Park.

H. Wilson, MD, PhD, MIL, Senior Lecturer in Pharmacology, University of Liverpool.

The scientific subcommittee

H. C. Gough, BSc, PhD, DIC, FIBiol (Chairperson), Lately Chief Science Specialist, Ministry of Agriculture, Fisheries and Food.

C. L. Berry, MD, PhD, FRCPath, Professor of Morbid Anatomy, The London Hospital Medical College; Hon. Consultant Pathologist, The London Hospital.

A. E. M. McLean, BM, BCh, PhD, MRCPath, Reader in Toxicology, Laboratory of Toxicology and Pharmacokinetics, University College Hospital, London.

F. M. Sullivan, BSc, Senior Lecturer in Pharmacology, Department of Pharmacology, Guys Hospital Medical School, London.

Appendix 11. Members of the Advisory Committee on Asbestos as of September 1979

W. J. Simpson (Chairperson), Chairperson, Health and Safety Commission.

E. D. Acheson, Dean, Faculty of Medicine, Southampton University, Professor of Clinical Epidemiology.

A. C. Blyghton, Secretary, Legal Department, Transport and General Workers Union.

P. Bradbury, Chairperson, CBI Safety, Health and Welfare Committee. Lately Personnel Director, Imperial Group Ltd.

J. C. Gilson, formerly Director, Medical Research Council, Pneumoconiosis Unit, Penarth.

H. D. S. Hardie, Director, Turner and Newall Ltd.

W. Lewis, Organisation Officer, Union of Construction Allied Trades and Technicians.

A. Lomas, National Union of Dyers, Bleachers and Textile Workers.

A. Mair, Professor of Community and Occupational Medicine, Dundee University.

M. Molyneux, Occupational Hygienist, Institute of Naval Medicine.

C. J. Stairmand, Consultant Chemical Engineer and Physicist.

J. Steel, Consultant to WHO in Industrial Hygiene; Senior Lecturer, Nuffield Department of Industrial Health, University of Newcastle-upon-Tyne; Consultant in Occupational Hygiene to the North of England Health Service.

F. G. Sugden, Chief Environmental Health Officer, Middlesborough.

M. Turner-Warwick, Professor of Medicine (Thoracic Medicine), University of London; Consultant to Brompton and London Chest Hospitals.

A. W. Ure, member CBI Safety and Health Panel; member of Royal Commission on Compensation for Personal Injury; director, Trollope and Colls Ltd.

R. Waterhouse, member of National Consumer Council, member of Council of Consumer Associations.

Appendix 12. Threshold Limit Values*

What are Threshold Limit Values?

The government, through the Health and Safety Executive, tries to limit the harmful effects of dust, fumes, radiation, etc., by limiting the amount of such hazards that workers can be exposed to. These limits are called 'control' or 'exposure' limits. Unfortunately, the UK has not had the resources or expertise to set these limits for more than a handful of toxic substances. Accordingly, the HSE borrows them from the USA. Each year, American experts employed by the government and industry sit down and look at the evidence on toxicity for each of about 600 substances, and, after balancing health effects against cost, they agree on their control limits. These are called 'Threshold Limit Values' (TLVs). They are published in the USA, and about a year later the HSE publish them in this country, in their Guidance Note, EH 15; a paragraph for British readers describes the few UK control limits that differ from those fixed for the USA. The limits are then used to control harmful dusts and fumes in all workplaces. The TLVs are not legal standards themselves, but are used as evidence to show that substances are likely to be 'injurious to health' (sec. 63 of the Factories Act), or that not everything that is 'reasonably practicable' is being done to protect workers' health (sec. 2 of the Health and Safety at Work Act).

How are dust, fumes, etc., in the workplace compared to TLVs?

The substances in the workplace environment have to be measured, and this is done by monitoring the atmosphere in the workers' breathing zone with instruments that measure how much dust or fume is present. **Dust** is divided into 'total dust' (all dust), and 'respirable dust' (those normally invisible particles less than 5 microns across which get right into the lungs)

---

* This appendix was originally issued as a briefing document by the Health and Safety Department of the GMWU.

and is usually measured with a portable pump and filter head. This draws air past the workers' mouth and nose area, deposits the dust particles on a filter which is then weighed. The amount of dust is then given in *milligrams per cubic metre or mg/m^3* for short. Respirable fibrous dusts like asbestos and glass fibre are measured in numbers of fibres per cubic centimetre of air, i.e. *fibres/cc*. **Fumes** are usually measured with gas detector tubes, which change colour like the breathaliser when particular fumes are present; or with portable pumps and filter beds that trap the fume. The fume is then analysed and the amount is given in either volume terms, i.e. *parts of the gas per million of air* (*ppm*), or sometimes in weight terms, i.e. *milligrams per cubic metre* (mg/m^3). Both 'ppm' and 'mg/m^3' results are different ways of measuring the same amount of gas. The monitoring has to be representative of what workers are breathing. The location, timing and duration of sampling is therefore crucial, and safety representatives and operators should be consulted about the monitoring.

The results of monitoring are then compared to the TLV, which may be described as a *Time Weighted Average* (TWA) or as a *Ceiling value* (C). The TWA is the *average* amount of the substance over the 8-hour day or shift to which workers may be exposed. High and low concentrations (i.e. amounts) of the substance during the day are balanced out, giving an average result which must be below the TWA. Very high concentrations of some substances, (e.g. carbon monoxide), would kill or harm workers, so these are limited by *Short-term Exposure Limits* (STEL), or *excursion factors*, which are described and listed in the TLV's list. Some substances can act very quickly, or can cause damage that cannot be reversed so balancing high concentrations against low concentrations is nonsense, and they must be kept below a 'C' limit all the time. These substances in the TLV list are marked with a 'C'.

How useful are TLVs?

TLVs can be useful: (i) in persuading management and workers that there could be a serious hazard at work if their workplace substance is listed (but there may still be a hazard if its not listed, see below); (ii) in providing a target figure for dirty workplaces to reach; and (iii) in providing a maximum upper limit to the levels which unions and safety representatives will allow in the cleaner workplaces. TLVs may seem to be very scientific and certain, but they are very rough guidelines that do not protect all workers. In general, safety representatives therefore should insist that all monitoring results are kept below half of the TLV (or below half the control limit recommended by the union) because of the following problems with TLVs.

What's wrong with TLVs?

(1) Only a few substances have TLVs – the rest are assumed to be safe. There are at least 60,000 chemicals in common use but only about 600 have been given TLVs. The rest are usually assumed to be 'safe' by employers, because there's no evidence to suggest that they are harmful. But 'no evidence' usually means that no one has looked for any. It is often the bodies of workers that finally provide the evidence of harm. Substances are therefore given the luxury of being 'safe' until proved harmful. We must reverse this process and assume substances are likely to be harmful, until proved 'safe' by experiments and medical checks. All substances should be regarded as toxic, and workplace exposures reduced to a minimum even if no TLV exists. Use a target figure of one-tenth of whatever is first measured at work if no TLV exists. Find out from your employer and the union what evidence of toxicity exists for your workplace substances, because reference books give evidence on at least 12,000 substances, even if most of these have no TLV.

(2) TLVs are based on the maximum acceptable levels of effect on workers, rather than on the minimum detectable change in the body's functions. The Americans define a TLV as the concentration of a substance to which it is *believed* that *nearly all* workers may be repeatedly exposed day after day without adverse *effect*. (We'll see below that the 'belief' may be based on poor evidence, and that some workers will not be protected by the TLV.) The 'effect' means no injury to health, or 'reasonable' freedom from irritation, feeling dizzy, nuisance or some other stress. But well before these effects are felt by workers, or diagnosed by doctors, the body's cells and functions will have been affected by the substance, and this can usually be measured with biological or psychological tests. Some scientists, especially in the USSR, consider that these first effects are likely to lead to some damage in the future, and so they fix the control limits at levels which do not allow any of these effects in workers. As a result, their control limits are much lower than the American TLVs. For example, about half the substances listed in the USA (and therefore in the UK) have TLVs that are 5 times higher than the Russian limits, and some have limits that are over 50 times higher.

(3) TLVs involve balancing the health effects against the costs of avoiding them. TLVs are fixed by experts who look at the evidence on health, then at the levels of the substance in workplaces, and then a limit is fixed which will not harm too many workers and will not cost employers too much. If substances have been thrown around the workplace like water then the evidence of harm would have to be massive if the TLV is to be fixed at a low level. Notice that workers who face the risks that the

experts consider acceptable are not usually consulted – neither in the USA or UK. This explains why other US health authorities like NIOSH and the GMWU often fix lower control limits than the American TLVs. For example, NIOSH and the GMWU recommend 25 ppm for trichloro-ethylene (instead of 100 ppm, as in the TLV list) and 35 ppm for carbon monoxide (instead of 50 ppm, as in the TLV list). The union accepts that some compromise between health and costs always has to be reached, but as representatives of the people that take the risks, we will usually want a better compromise than 'experts' give us.

(4) TLVs are based on average workers, and no worker is average. First, the little research that has been done on workers has usually involved people whose health is above average, often young, fit, white males. Workers are not always like that. Women, other races, and younger or older people may be more or less sensitive to substances. And, second, all workers are different even within a group of fit, 25-year-old, white males because their biological make up is different. This means that the same dose of a substance will have a different effect on different individuals, e.g. we will not all die from lung cancer after smoking 20 cigarettes a day – only some of us will. The experts who fix the TLVs admit this and say 'a small percentage of workers may experience discomfort from some substances at or below TLV; a smaller percentage may be affected more seriously by aggravation of a pre-existing condition, or by development of an occupational illness.' These 'small' groups of workers can be large. A study of 90 substances and their TLVs showed that 50 per cent of workers will be affected by irritant materials at the TLV level, 4 per cent will be affected by narcotic materials (e.g. solvents that make you drowsy), 20 per cent will suffer some damage to health, and 1 in 10,000 will die at the TLV level.

Finally, if the substance causes 'sensitisation', like TDI, then, once sensitised, workers will react to almost any level. Workers sensitised to TDI have reacted with asthmatic coughing, etc., to concentrations that were less than one-twentieth of the TLV.

(5) TLVs are based on inadequate research. TLVs are often fixed on very little evidence, or on evidence about the acute, or short-term effects of the substance. Only about 20 per cent of the substances listed are based on any evidence about their chronic, or long-term effects. For example, although it is accepted that all dusts cause some effect on the lungs after a time, the TLV for those dusts – called 'nuisance dusts' – is based on the view that you cannot *see* when the dust in the workplace is above 10 mg/m^3! More research would probably cause TLVs to fall faster than they do now. Much of the evidence that is used comes from the effects of high doses, and no one knows what the effect of low doses might be. For

example, people 'guess' what the effects of low-level radiation might be on the evidence from the Japanese atomic bombs and other high level doses, but there is evidence to suggest that this will underestimate the risks of low doses.

(6) TLVs are based on the effect of one substance at a time – most workers are exposed to many. No one knows what the effects of several substances together might be, but it is likely that many substances react with each other to produce effects that are accumulatively far worse than the sum of their parts. For example, smoking and asbestos increases the risks by much more than the risks of each added to each other. When radon gas found in non-coal mines gets absorbed onto dust particles and carried into the lung, its toxic effect increases by 30 times. And when nitrogen oxides, found after blasting or in diesel exhaust fumes, attach themselves to fairly harmless dust particles, their toxicity doubles. One study found that 5 per cent of toxic substances behave in this way. The TLVs assume that all substances just have the adding effect, which means they offer no protection at all against multiplying effects. Even so, the guidelines on 'mixtures' in the TLV list mean that each of several substances can be well below their separate TLVs, but the mixture together can be greater than the TLV for the mixture. For example, if three substances are measured, and they are four-tenths of the TLV, three-quarters of the TLV and one-half of the TLV, respectively, then their combined concentration is well above the TLV for the mixture. ($0.4 + 0.75 + 0.5 = 1.65$, when anything above 1.0 exceeds the TLV).

(7) Substances can add to the effects of other harmful agents at work, like noise; or with non-work substances, like alcohol, medicines, etc; the TLVs do not allow for this. Workers are subject to noise, heat, radiation, etc., and toxic substances can combine with these to produce more harmful effects than they would by themselves. For example, noise and some chemicals that damage the nervous system, like carbon monoxide and trichloro-ethylene ('trike'), can make the effect of the noise or the chemical on hearing worse than if just the noise or the chemical was present. 'Trike' when present at the same time as heat from welding decomposes and give off the highly poisonous phosgene gas. PTFE can be broken down by smoking, giving off a more deadly substance. And because a worker's body is dealing with toxic substances from work, it has greater problems with chemicals absorbed at home. For example, alcohol and 'trike' can cause flushing and reddening in the face; and rubber workers found that their bodies did not get rid of the toxic residues from hydrogen sulphide after work if they were also taking headache tablets. The worst example is between smoking and some dusts. The TLVs

provide hardly any protection against these reactions with other harmful agents.

(8) TLVs are based on 'normal' workplaces and a 40-hour week. If workers are exposed to extremes of temperature (e.g. above 90°F); or if they work more than 50 hours a week; or if they are subjected to unusual air pressure or humidity, then even without the multiplying reactions described above, these additional stresses on the body are likely to make substances more harmful. The TLVs do not allow for these 'gross variations' in the workers' environment. So regular overtime (over 10 hours a week) damages health as well as depressing basic wages.

(9) TLVs are based on the inhalation route only – they do not protect against absorption through the skin, or ingestion. Substances can enter the body through three routes – through the nose and mouth (inhalation), through the skin (absorption) and through the stomach (ingestion). Many substances can enter via all three routes, but the TLVs are based on the inhalation route only. A substance in the list is marked with the word 'skin' if it can also enter that way. Full eye and skin protection is then needed, or a lower TLV must be used.

(10) Monitoring the working atmosphere gives only a rough guide to what workers are really exposed to. In trying to find out whether workers are exposed to concentrations of substances above the TLVs, the working atmosphere is monitored. However, there is a good chance that errors will be made due to: (i) random variations in the working environment both within one day, and from day to day; (ii) other variations in the environment due to open doors, faulty ventilation, or changed production conditions; and (iii) error in the sampling and analysing instruments and methods. *This means that just grabbing a sample of air with a gas detector tube can give no assurance that workers are getting less than the TLV*. Only continuous monitoring for 8 hours, or the full shift every day, with allowances (say 10 per cent) for instrument and techniques error, can approach this guarantee. However, if monitoring is done regularly (with workers consultation on where, when and for how long), then, as long as all results are kept below half of the TLV or other recommended control limit, there's a reasonable guarantee that workers are not being exposed to concentrations above the TLV.

The GMWU briefing document reprinted above shows that TLVs are often set on the flimsiest of data and reflect industrial pressure and convenience of current practice far more than any objective assessment of the evidence. The Health and Safety Executive admitted this in a confidential document issued in early 1982, stating that 'the TLVs are set unilaterally by the ACGIH and sometimes not obviously on the basis of medical data' (see *Health and Safety at Work*, March 1982, p. 17). The HSE, therefore, intends to abandon TLVs and to adopt so called 'control limits' instead. Whereas TLVs purport to be based principally on medical evidence, control limits have no such pretensions. No level is presumed 'safe' and the control limit would explicitly take notice of what the relevant industry see as economically feasible, or, in the language of the HSE, what is supposed to be 'reasonably practicable'. Such a procedure explicitly involves the trading off of the costs of stricter control of a dangerous material against the costs, in death and disability, of chemically-induced cancers and other diseases. The control limit would supposedly be set at a point which minimises these two costs and could presumably be reduced further as the costs of control are reduced by technical progress.

The control limits scheme has considerable deficiencies. If the standards to be drawn up imply an assessment of trade-offs between medical evidence and the costs of control, then it is vital that the inevitable claims of companies that they cannot afford stricter controls should be open to public scrutiny and criticism. Also, it is vital that the methods by which the trade-off is to be made are publicly debated. This is unlikely, given the HSE's commitment to maintaining confidentiality and commercial secrecy. In fact, neither TLV nor control limits provide an adequate basis for reducing exposure to carcinogens in the workplace, particularly where the system of enforcement is so weak.

Notes

Place of publication is London unless stated otherwise.

1. The politics of cancer

1. S. Sontag, *Illness as Metaphor*, New York, Vintage Books (1979).
2. See Peto's discussion in appendix 2.
3. For a summary of his position, see appendix 3.
4. ASTMS, *The Prevention of Occupational Cancer* (1980); GMWU, *A Preliminary Cancer Prevention Campaign* (1980); NGA, *Occupational Cancer in the Printing Industry* (1980). For details of where to obtain these, see appendix 6.
5. The most significant recent example of these are reproduced as appendices 2 and 3.
6. ASTMS, *The Prevention of Occupational Cancer* (1980); CIA, *Cancer in Modern Mortality* (1980); J. Keir Howard, *The Prevention of Occupational Cancer: A Review*, CIA (1980).
7. Report of an IARC Working Group, *Cancer Research*, vol. 40, no. 1 (1980).
8. J. Robinson, 'Cervical cancer: a feminist critique', *Times Health Supplement*, 27 November 1981; J. Robinson, 'Cancer of the cervix: occupational risks of husbands and wives and possible preventive strategies, Proceedings of the Ninth Study Group of the Royal College of Obstetricians and Gynaecologists, RCOG, 1982.
9. D. Forman, 'The Politics of Cancer', *Marxism Today*, August 1981.

2. The cancer problem

1. T. McKeown, R. G. Record and R. D. Turner, 'An interpretation of the decline in mortality in England and Wales during the twentieth century', *Population Studies*, 29 (1975), pp. 391–422.
2. *Mortality Statistics: Cause 1980*, series DH2 no. 7, OPCS (1982).
3. For the American data, see S. Epstein, *The Politics of Cancer*, New York, Anchor Press (1979), chapter 1; for British data, see *Cancer*

Statistics: Survival 1971–73 Registrations, series MBI no. 3, OPCS
(1980). See also D. Gould, 'Cancer – a conspiracy of silence', *New
Scientist*, 2 December 1976, pp. 522–23.

4. *Trends in Mortality 1951–75*, series DH1 no. 3, OPCS (1978).

5. *Ibid.*

6. *Ibid.*

7. *Ibid.*

8. For a discussion of this evidence, see Epstein, *Politics of Cancer*,
   pp. 14–16.

9. The best source of evidence for these differences is *Occupational
   Mortality: The Registrar General's Decennial Supplement for England
   and Wales, 1970–72*, series DS no. 1, OPCS (1978). This is the most
   recent in a series of reports provided at ten-year intervals.

10. The Standardised Mortality Ratio (SMR) is the percentage ratio of
    the number of deaths observed in a specific group studied to the
    number that would be expected from the age-specific death rates for
    the total population of England and Wales.

11. This refers to the five 'social class' categories often used in the
    presentation of British official statistics. The categories are based on
    occupation, social class I being the 'highest' (professional and
    managerial) and social class V the 'lowest' (unskilled).

12. There is a useful discussion of this in *Occupational Mortality*. See
    also, A. J. Fox and A. M. Adelstein, 'Occupational mortality: work
    or way of life?', *Journal of Epidemiology and Community Health*, 32
    (1978), pp. 73–78.

13. For a more detailed discussion of this point and its relationship to
    health issues, see L. Doyal with I. Pennell, *The Political Economy of
    Health*, Pluto Press (1979), chapter 2.

14. For a detailed account of this evidence, see appendix 3.

15. ASTMS, *The Prevention of Occupational Cancer* (1980), p. 55.

16. These figures are published annually by the Department of Health
    and Social Security.

17. See letters to the *New Statesman* by R. Peto, 10 September 1982, and
    D. Gee, 1 October 1982.

18. ASTMS, *Prevention of Occupational Cancer*, p. 17.

19. J. Robinson, 'Cervical cancer: a feminist critique', *Times Health
    Supplement*, 27 November 1981.

20. For a discussion of these trends see B. Jacobson, *The Ladykillers:
    Why Smoking is a Feminist Issue*, Pluto Press (1981), and S.
    Stellman and J. Stellman, 'Women's occupations, smoking, cancer
    and other diseases', *Cancer Journal for Clinicians*, 31 (1981),
    pp. 29–41.

21. Doyal with Pennell, *Political Economy of Health*, pp. 83–92; Politics of Health Group, Pamphlet no. 1, *Food and Profit* (1979); C. Wardle, *Changing Food Habits in the UK: An Assessment of the Social, Technological, Economic and Political Factors which Influence Dietary Patterns*, Friends of the Earth (1977).
22. For a summary of these developments see: Boston Women's Health Book Collective, *Our Bodies Ourselves: A Health Book by and for Women*, British edition by A. Phillips and J. Rakusen, Harmondsworth, Penguin (1978).
23. P. Stocks, 'On the relations between atmospheric pollution in urban and rural localities', *British Journal of Cancer*, 14 (1960), pp. 397–418.
24. S. S. Epstein, L. O. Brown and C. Pope, *Hazardous Waste in America*, Sierra Club Books, San Francisco (1982).
25. O. L. Lloyd, 'Respiratory cancer clustering associated with localised industrial air pollution', *Lancet*, 1 (1978), pp. 318–20.
26. M. J. Gardner, P. D. Winter, E. D. Acheson, 'Variations in cancer mortality among local authority areas in England and Wales: relations with environmental factors and search for causes', *British Medical Journal*, 284 (1982), pp. 784–87.

3. How carcinogens are controlled

1. *Chemical and Engineering News*, 9 June 1980.
2. J. Walsh, 'EPA and toxic substances law: dealing with uncertainty', *Science*, 202 (1978), pp. 598–602; Health and Safety Executive, *Proposed Scheme for the Notification of Toxic Properties of Substances* (1977).
3. See appendix 7 for a list of those organisations which do exist in fields related to the fight against cancer.
4. Office of Science and Technology, Council on Environmental Quality Ad Hoc Committee, *Report on Environmental Health Research* (Washington, DC, June 1972), quoted in S. Epstein, *The Politics of Cancer*, New York, Anchor Press (1979), p. 321.
5. NIEHS, *Report to the Senate Appropriation Committee on Federal Support for Environmental Health Research* (1977), quoted in Epstein, *Politics of Cancer*, p. 321.
6. *Fortune*, 13 February 1978, p. 116.
7. Medical Research Council, *Annual Report* (1978–79).
8. Royal Society, *Long-term Hazards to Man from Man-made Chemicals in the Environment* (1978), quoted in 'Royal Society slams routine toxicity tests', *Nature*, 274 (1978), p. 413.

9. The first major legislation of this sort was the Factory Act of 1833. See K. Marx, *Capital*, vol. 1, Harmondsworth, Penguin (1976), pp. 389–416.

10. The most recent moves in this campaign are discussed in G. Wilson *et al.*, *Cancer at work: Dyes*, Cancer Prevention Society (1980) (for address of the society see appendix 7). See also new HSE Guidance Note, *Health and Safety Precautions for Benzidine-based Dyes*, EH/34 (August 1982).

11. Health and Safety Executive, *Toxic Substances: A Precautionary Policy*, note EH18 (1977).

12. H. J. Dunster, *Carcinogens in the Workplace*, Technical Report, Health and Safety Executive (1982).

13. Quoted in the *Guardian*, 1 March 1982.

14. *Chemistry and Industry*, 15 April 1978, p. 504.

15. 'Chemical company suppresses dioxin report', *Nature* 284 (1980), p. 2. ASTMS, *Report on Coalite Chemicals*, May 1980.

16. *Official Journal of the European Community*, no. L 259/10, 15 October 1979.

17. *European Chemical News*, 8 January 1979, p. 19, and 2 July 1979, p. 17.

18. ASTMS, *The Prevention of Occupational Cancer* (1980), p. 52.

19. Health and Safety Executive, *Toxic Substances: A Precautionary Policy*.

20. Health and Safety Commission, *Notification of New Substances*, consultative document, HMSO (1981).

21. The Nightwear (Safety) Order (1978), and the Balloon-making Compounds (Safety) Order (1979), respectively.

22. These relate to the emission of hydrochloric acid gas from alkali works, to sulphuric acid works and to muriatic acid works.

23. This list is taken from Department of Environment Central Unit on Environmental Pollution, *Pollution Control in Great Britain – How it Works*, Pollution Paper no. 9, HMSO (1978), pp. 86–89.

24. See Health and Safety Executive, *Lists of Registrable Works and Noxious or Offensive Gases Specified in the Acts and Orders* (1977).

25. Royal Commission on Environmental Pollution, Fifth Report, *Air Pollution Control: An Integrated Approach*, HMSO (1976), p. 24.

26. Quoted in M. Frankel, *The Alkali Inspectorate*, Social Audit (1974), p. 8.

27. H.M. Chief Inspector of Factories, *Annual Report 1972*, HMSO (1973).

28. Frankel, *The Alkai Inspectorate*, p. 27.

29. Royal Commission on Environmental Pollution, Fifth Report, *Air Pollution Control*, pp. 33–4.

4. Case studies: the workplace

1. Figures given in reply to a written parliamentary question from Dr O. McDonald, MP, 27 October 1980, *Hansard*, vol. 991, HMSO (1980).
2. *Times* 28 March 1977; figures supplied by the Asbestos Information Centre.
3. M. Greenberg and T. A. Lloyd Davis, 'Mesothelioma register, 1967–68', *British Journal of Industrial Medicine*, 31 (1974), pp. 91–104; A. Dalton, *Asbestos: Killer Dust*, British Society for Social Responsibility in Science (1979).
4. M. L. Newhouse, 'A study of the mortality of workers in an asbestos factory', *British Journal of Industrial Medicine*, 26 (1969), pp. 294–301.
5. Figures given in reply to a written parliamentary question from Mr D. Skinner, MP, 5 June 1980, *Hansard*, vol. 985, HMSO (1980).
6. Letters by R. Peto and D. Gee to *New Statesman*, 10 September and 1 October 1982.
7. Parliamentary Commissioner for Administration, *Third Report*, HMSO (1976).
8. *Journal of the Royal College of Physicians*, 12 (1978), p. 297.
9. W. Burton Wood and F. Roodhouse Gloyne, 'Pulmonary asbestosis: a review of 100 cases', *Lancet*, 2 (1934), pp. 1383–85.
10. Committee on Hygiene Standards of British Occupational Hygiene Society, 'Hygiene standards for chrysotile asbestos dust', *Annals of Occupational Hygiene*, 11 (1968), p. 47. By 'asbestosis' the committee meant the earliest demonstrable effect on the lungs due to asbestos.
11. H. Lewinsohn, 'The medical surveillance of asbestos workers', *Journal of the Royal Society of Health*, 2 (1972), pp. 69–73.
12. Dalton, *Asbestos: Killer Dust*, p. 122.
13. S. A. Roach, 'Hygiene standards for asbestos', *Annals of Occupational Hygiene*, 13 (1970), pp. 7–15.
14. Advisory Committee on Asbestos (Health and Safety Commission), *Asbestos: Final Report*, HMSO (1979), para. 127.
15. J. Peto, 'The hygiene standard for chrysotile asbestos', *Lancet*, 1 (1978), pp. 484–89.
16. R. Peto and D. Gee, letters to the *New Statesman*, 10 September and 1 October 1982.
17. See ASTMS, 'Health hazards of man-made fibres', *Monitor* no. 12 (July 1981), and *The Hazards of Glass Fibre and Rockwool*, GMWU News Service, August 1982.

18. Quoted in R. Hudspith, 'The use of benzene in laboratories', unpublished MSc thesis, University of Manchester (1979).

19. ASTMS, *The Prevention of Occupational Cancer* (1980), p. 43; emphasis in original.

20. GMWU, *Hazard-Benzene* (1979).

21. R. J. Fielden, 'Review of toxicology of benzene', EMAS C4 (September 1980), unpublished.

22. The review devoted considerable space to a recent Dow study that reports increased mortality from leukaemia amongst workers exposed to benzene levels of less than 10 ppm. It notes that three deaths from leukaemia, besides two deaths from anaemia, were recorded (out of 549 workers), against an expected number of 0.8. However, the review refuses to accept this as evidence, on the grounds that no detailed medical history of the three workers is given. They all had a varied background and no cases of leukaemia were recorded amongst workers with higher levels of exposure. The Dow study is reported in M. G. Ott *et al.*, *Archives of Environmental Health*, vol. 33 (1978), pp. 3–10.

23. 'Supreme Court's divided benzene decision preserves uncertainty over regulation of environmental carcinogens', *Environmental Law Reporter*, 10 (1980), pp. 1192–8.

24. R. A. Rinsky *et al.*, 'Leukemia in benzene workers', *American Journal of Industrial Medicine*, 2 (1981), pp. 217–45.

25. *Financial Times*, 18 June 1982.

26. D. Russell, 'The role of the Chemical Industries Association in the regulation of the vinyl chloride monomer hazard', unpublished MSc thesis, University of Manchester (1979).

27. P. Viola, 'Carcinogenic effects of vinyl chloride', *Proceedings of the Tenth International Cancer Conference*, Houston (1970).

28. C. Maltoni, 'Occupational carcinogenesis: New facts, priorities and perspectives', *IARC Scientific Publication*, no. 13 (1976), Lyon. See also Epstein, *The Politics of Cancer*, pp. 104–7.

29. Chemical Industries Association, *CISHEC – The Chemical Industry Safety and Health Council*, CIA Publications (undated), p. 16.

30. C. Clutterbuck, 'Death in the plastics factory', *Radical Science Journal*, no. 4 (1976), pp. 61–80.

31. D. Russell, 'Role of the CIA in the regulation of the VCM hazard'.

32. A. W. Barnes, 'National and international aspects of the VC problems', *BFF/PRI Joint Conference*, part II, May 1975, p. 13.

33. MAFF, *Steering Group on Food Surveillance: Second Report*, HMSO (1978).

34. HSE, *Report on Industrial Air Pollution, 1976,* HMSO (1978), pp. 14–15.

35. *Ibid.*
36. See S. Epstein, *The Politics of Cancer*, New York, Anchor Press (1979), p. 114.
37. *Official Journal of The European Community*, no. L197, 22 February 1978, pp. 12–18.
38. *Industrial Relations Review and Report*, October 1980.
39. *Ibid.*
40. IARC, *Monograph on Evaluation of the Carcinogenic Risk of Chemicals to Humans*, vol. 19, February 1979, p. 417.
41. Chemical Industries Association, *Acrylonitrile Status Report*, 1 June 1977.
42. S. Epstein, *The Politics of Cancer*, p. 211.
43. 'Panorama', BBC TV, 5 June 1978.
44. *Ibid.*
45. MAFF, Steering Group on Food Surveillance, *Survey of Acrylonitrile: Food Surveillance Paper 6*, HMSO (1981).
46. W. C. Bauman, Physical Research Laboratory (1948) for Dow Chemical, quoted in the company's submission on BCME to US Department of Labor, May 1973.
47. W. G. Figueroa, R. Raszkowski and W. Weiss, 'Lung cancer in chloromethyl ether workers', *New England Journal of Medicine*, 288 (1973), pp. 1096–97. Epstein maintains that some 14 cases had already been identified by 1962. S. Epstein, *The Politics of Cancer*, Anchor Press (1979), p. 119.
48. Dow Chemical Company's submission on BCME to US Department of Labor, p. 4.
49. B. L. van Duuren *et al.*, 'Alpha-haloethers – a new type of alkylating carcinogen', *Archives of Environmental Health*, vol. 16 (April 1968).
50. J. L. Gargus *et al.*, 'Induction of lung adenomas in new-born mice by BisCME', *Toxicology and Applied Pharmacology*, 15–92–6 (1969).
51. Figueroa *et al.*, 'Lung cancer in chloromethyl ether workers'.
52. Report by Dr Murray, 'Chemicals and cancer', letter to GMWU, 31 October 1969.
53. S. Laskin *et al.*, 'Tumours of the respiratory tract induced by inhalation of BisCME', *Archives of Environmental Health*, vol. 23 (August 1971), pp. 135–36.
54. K. J. Leong *et al.*, 'Induction of lung adenomas by chronic inhalation of BisCME', *Archives of Environmental Health*, vol. 22 (June 1971), pp. 663–660.
55. S. Laskin *et al.*, 'Inhalation carcinogenicity of alpha-haloethers', paper presented to British occupational Hygiene Society's Fourth International Symposium (1971).

56. Dr Norton Nelson, leader of the New York team of Norton, Laskin, van Duuren *et al.*, had used federal funds to study BCME after losing the animal-testing contract to Hazelton Laboratories in 1966. Reported by N. S. Randall and S. D. Solomon, '94 who died', *Philadelphia Inquirer*, 26 October 1975.

57. Dr Murray's report to GMWU, December 1971.

58. Dr Murray's report to GMWU, 23 June 1972.

59. 'Chemical suspected in 6 cases of lung cancer', *Occupational Health and Safety Letter*, 2.6.72, cited in Figueroa *et al.*, 'Lung cancer in chloromethyl ether workers'.

60. L. R. Defonso and S. C. Kelton, 'Lung cancer following exposure to CME', *Archives of Environmental Health*, vol. 31 (May–June 1976), pp. 125–30.

61. Dr Murray's report to GMWU, 23 June 1972.

62. Figueroa *et al.*, 'Lung cancer in chloromethyl ether workers'.

63. Following the NIOSH study at the Diamond Shamrock Plant, the human evidence of the carcinogenicity of BCME was confirmed in J. K. Wagoner, 'Carcinogenicity of BisCME', paper presented at ACGIH conference, Boston. 1973. A. M. Thiess *et al.*, 'Toxicology of BisCME – suspicion of carcinogenicity in man', *Zentralbl. Arbeitsmedizin*, vol. 23 (1973), pp. 97–102. H. Sakabe, 'Lung cancer due to BisCME', *Industrial Health*, vol. 11 (August 1973). This reported 5 cases among 32 workers exposed to BCME in a Japanese dyestuffs factory.

64. R. I. McCallum, Report on the carcinogenicity of BisCME and CME at Permutit Factory, Pontyclun, Glamorgan (April 1973).

65. Letter from Dr. T. V. Arden, Director, Water Research Centre, to GMWU, 19 May 1981.

66. Dow Chemical submission on BCME to US Dept. of Labor, 1973.

67. Letter from Dr K. Duncan, to GMWU, 21 August 1980.

68. R. A. Lemen *et al.*, 'Cytologic observations and cancer incidence following exposure to BisCME', in U. Saffiotti and J. K. Wagoner (eds), *Occupational Carcinogenesis, Annals of New York Academy of Sciences*, vol. 271 (1976) pp. 71–80. Defonso and Kelton, 'Lung cancer following exposure to CME', reported excess lung cancer rates at the Rohm and Haas plant in the US.

69. Letter from Dr K. Howard of the Chemical Industries Association to Diamond Shamrock, 3 April 1980.

70. McCallum *et al.*, 'Lung cancer associated with chloromethyl ether manufacture: an investigation of two factories in the UK', preliminary report, 1982. No excess was found at the Newcastle factory of Rohm and Haas.

5. Case studies: consumer products

1. Royal College of Physicians, *Smoking and Health Now*, Pitman Medical (1971), p. 9.
2. *Mortality Statistics 1979. England and Wales*, series DH1 no. 8, OPCS (1982). See also Appendix 3.
3. Royal College of Physicians, *Smoking or Health?*, Pitman Medical (1977).
4. T. Hirayama, 'Non-smoking wives of heavy smokers have a higher risk of lung cancer: a study from Japan', *British Medical Journal*, 282 (1981), pp. 183–85.
5. Royal College of Physicians, *Smoking and Health Now*, p. 33.
6. *Ibid.* pp. 95–6.
7. *General Household Survey 1980*, OPCS (1981).
8. *Ibid.*
9. *Ibid.*
10. *Ibid.* See also, G. F. Todd, *Social Class Variations in Tobacco Smoking and in Mortality from Associated Diseases*, Occasional Paper no. 2, Tobacco Research Council (1978); and J. Townsend, 'Smoking and class', *New Society*, 30 March 1978, pp. 709–10.
11. *Times Health Supplement*, 27 November 1981, p. 3.
12. See also an interesting article by P. N. Lee, 'Has the mortality of male doctors improved with the reduction in their cigarette smoking?', *British Medical Journal*, 2 (1979), pp. 1538–40.
13. Y. Bostock, B. Jacobson, P. White and L. Seymour, 'Ad-man's bull's-eye – researcher's blank', *The Health Services*, 9 June 1982. For a detailed treatment of women and smoking, see B. Jacobson, *The Ladykillers: Why Smoking is a Feminist Issue*, Pluto Press (1981).
14. Bostock *et al.*, 'Ad-man's bull's-eye – researcher's blank'.
15. *Ibid.*
16. Jacobson, *The Ladykillers*.
17. ASH, *The Economics of Smoking*, Fact Sheet no. 3. Available from Action on Smoking and Health (ASH), 27–35 Mortimer Street, London W1N 7RJ.
18. C. Hird, 'Taking on the tobacco man', *New Statesman*, 27 February 1981.
19. *Ibid.*
20. N. Wood, *Times Health Supplement*, 12 March 1982, p. 6.
21. *Ibid.* See also letter from Dr Brian Lloyd to *Times Health Supplement*, 19 March 1982.
22. N. Wood, *Times Health Supplement*, 12 March 1982.

23. Lloyd, letter to *Times Health Supplement*, 19 March 1982.

24. M. Dean, 'Blowing away smoke screens', *Guardian*, 4 January 1980.

25. M. Muller, *Tobacco and the Third World: Tomorrow's Epidemic?*, War on Want (1978).

26. ASH, *The Economics of Smoking*.

27. *New Scientist*, 14 August 1975, p. 369.

28. 'Medical charities and prevention', *British Medical Journal*, 22 December 1979, p. 1610. For an extremely interesting discussion of the bias in cancer research, see R. W. Moss, *The Cancer Syndrome*, New York, Grove Press (1982).

29. R. Kinosita, 'Studies on the carcinogenic azo and related compounds', *Yale Journal of Biology and Medicine*, 12 (1940), p. 287.

30. W. Schiller, *American Journal of Cancer*, 31 (1937), pp. 486–90.

31. A. H. M. Kirby and P. R. Peacock, 'Liver tumours in mice injected with commercial food dyes', *Glasgow Medical Journal*, 30 (1949), pp. 364–70.

32. Food Standards Committee, *Report on Colouring Matters*, HMSO (1954), para. 43.

33. P. R. Peacock, 'Colouring matter in foods', *Chemistry and Industry*, 15 March 1952, pp. 238–41.

34. *The Colouring Matter in Food Regulations*, Statutory Instrument no. 1,066 (1957).

35. M. M. Andrianova, *Voprosij Pitaniya*, vol. 29 no. 5 (1970), p. 61.

36. S. Epstein, *The Politics of Cancer*, New York, Anchor Press (1979), pp. 183–85.

37. Departmental Committee on Preservatives and Colouring Matters in Food, *Final Report*, HMSO (1924).

38. Food Additives and Contaminants Committee, *Interim Report on the Review of the Colouring Matter in Food Regulations 1973*, HMSO (1979).

39. Food Standards Committee, *Report on Food Colours*, HMSO (1954).

40. Food Standards Committee, *Report on Food Colours*, HMSO (1964).

41. 'Significance of recent studies on amaranth', *BIBRA Bulletin*, vol. 10 no. 28 (1971). BIBRA is a toxicological testing institution funded by industry and government. See S. Epstein, *The Politics of Cancer*, pp. 311–12.

42. Committee on the Toxicity of Chemicals in Food, Consumer Products and the Environment, *Report on the Review of the*

Colouring Matter in Food Regulations 1973, Annex 2 in Food Additives and Contaminants Committee, *Interim Report*, HMSO (1979).

43. S. Epstein, *The Politics of Cancer*, p. 185.

44. B. Armstrong and R. Doll, Bladder cancer mortality in England and Wales in relation to cigarette smoking and saccharin consumption', *British Journal of Preventive and Social Medicine*, 28 (1974), pp. 233–40.

45. J. M. Price *et al.*, 'Bladder tumours in rats fed cyclohexylamine or high doses of cyclamate and saccharine', *Science*, 167 (1970), pp. 1131–32. B. L. Oser *et al.*, *Toxicology*, 6 (1975), pp. 47–65.

46. Wisconsin Alumni Research Foundation Institute, *Preliminary Report Chronic Toxicity Study – Sodium Saccharin*, WARF, Madison, Wisconsin (1972).

47. D. L. Arnold *et al.*, 'Canadian saccharin study', *Science*, 197 (1977), p. 320.

48. Evidence given to FDA by C. J. Kokoski 3 May 1977 (see Epstein, *The Politics of Cancer*, pp. 193–7).

49. R. M. Hicks, J. J. Wakefield and J. Chowaniec, 'Co-carcinogenic action of saccharin in the chemical induction of bladder cancer', *Nature*, 243 (1973), pp. 347–49.

50. *Daily Express*, 11 March 1977.

51. *Daily Telegraph*, 11 March 1977.

52. Food Additives and Contaminants Committee, *Report on the Review of Sweeteners in Food*, HMSO (1982), para. 3.

53. Editorial, 'Sweet Reason', *Lancet*, 1 (1977), p. 634.

54. B. Armstrong and R. Doll, 'Bladder cancer mortality in diabetics in relation to saccharin consumption and smoking habits', *British Journal of Preventive and Social Medicine*, 29 (1975), pp. 73–81. B. Armstrong *et al.*, 'Cancer mortality and saccharin consumption in diabetics, *British Journal of Preventive and Social Medicine*, 30 (1976), pp. 151–57.

55. Editorial, *New Scientist*, 17 March 1977.

56. e.g. *Morning Star*, 11 March 1977.

57. M. Hicks and J. Chowaniec, 'American ban on saccharin', *British Medical Journal*, 1 (1977), p. 771.

58. G. R. Howe *et al.*, 'Artificial sweeteners and human bladder cancer', *Lancet*, 2 (1977), pp. 578–81.

59. Editorial, *Lancet*, 2 (1977), p. 592.

60. Letter from A. B. Miller and G. R. Howe, *Lancet*, 2 (1977), pp. 1221–22.

61. Epstein, *The Politics of Cancer*, pp. 197–98.

62. *Ibid.*, p. 191; M. B. McCann *et al.*, 'Non-caloric sweeteners and weight reduction', *Journal of the American Dietetics Association*, 32 (1956), pp. 327–30; National Academy of Sciences, Institute of Medicine, Committee on Saccharin, *Sweeteners: Issues and Uncertainties,* Washington (1975).

63. Office of Technology Assessment, *Cancer Testing Technology and Saccharin*, USGPO, Washington (1977).

64. 'EEC recommends saccharin controls', *New Scientist*, 18 May 1978.

65. Food Additives and Contaminants Committee, *Report on the Review of Sweeteners in Food*, HMSO (1982), para. 3.

66. E. Boyland, 'Saccharin: from carcinogen to promoter', *Nature*, 278 (1979), pp. 123–24.

67. Food Additives and Contaminants Committee, *Report on the Review of Sweeteners in Food*, HMSO (1982).

68. *Ibid.*, p. 28.

69. *Ibid.*, pp. 11–12.

70. P. N. Magee, R. Montesano and R. Preussman, 'N-nitroso compounds and related carcinogens', in C. E. Searle (ed.), *Chemical Carcinogens*, ACS, Washington (1976).

71. J. Sander, 'Information on carcinogenic nitroso compounds under biological conditions', in *Environment and Cancer*, Williams and Wilkins, Baltimore (1972).

72. W. Lijinsky and S. S. Epstein, 'Nitrosamines as environmental carcinogens', *Nature*, 225 (1970), p. 21.

73. *Public Health (Preservatives etc. in Food) Regulations* 1925, Schedule 1.

74. British Food Manufacturers' Research Association, *Food Research Report*, no. 3, August 1927, pp. 5–6.

75. British Food Manufacturers' Research Association, *Food Research Report*, no. 6, January 1929, p. 11.

76. *Ibid*.

77. BFMRA, *Food Research Report*, no. 40, January 1941.

78. Food Standards Committee, *Report on Preservatives in Food*, HMSO (1959); *Supplementary Report,* HMSO (1960).

79. *Preservatives in Food Regulations*, Statutory Instrument no. 1532 (1962).

80. H. Druckrey *et al., Arzneimittel Forschung*, 13 (1963), p.320.

81. J. Sakshang *et al.*, 'Dimethyl-nitrosamine; its hepatoxic effect in sheep and its occurrence in toxic batches of herring meal', *Nature* 206 (1965), p. 1261. Food Additives and Contaminants Committee, *Report on the Review of the Preservatives in Food Regulations 1962,* HMSO (1972), para. 84.

82. C. L. Cutting, *Safety of Cured Meat Products*, letter to the meat members of British Food Manufacturing Industries Research Association, 2 August 1966.

83. *Ibid*. Our emphasis.

84. P. N. Magee and J. M. Barnes, 'The production of malignant primary hepatic tumours in the rat, by feeding dimethyl-nitrosamine', *British Journal of Cancer*, 10 (1956), pp. 114–22.

85. Editorial, *Lancet*, 1 (1968), p. 1971.

86. FACC, *Report 1962*, para. 85.

87. R. Montesano and P. N. Magee, 'Metabolism of dimethyl-nitrosamine by human liver slices in vitro', *Nature*, 228 (1970).

88. Food Additives and Contaminants Committee, *Interim Report*, unpublished (1971), referred to in FACC, *Report on Preservatives 1967*, para. 86.

89. *Preservatives in Food (Amendment) Regulations 1971*, Statutory Instrument no. 882.

90. Committee on Medical Aspects of Food Policy, Pharmacology Subcommittee, *Report on Preservatives in Food* (1971). Published as annex 1 to FACC, *Report on Preservatives* (1972).

91. *Ibid*.

92. 'Environmental nitrosamines' *Lancet*, 2 (1973), pp. 1243–44.

93. T. A. Crough *et al*., 'An examination of some foodstuffs for the presence of volatile nitrosamines', *Journal of the Science of Food and Agriculture*, 28 (1977), pp. 345–51.

94. S. J. Butler, 'USDA's role and plans regarding the use of nitrites in cured meats', *Food Technology*, 34 (1980), pp. 252–53.

95. P. Newberne, 'Nitrite promotes lymphoma incidence in rat', *Science*, 204, (1979), pp. 1079–81.

96. S. A. Miller, 'Balancing the risks regarding the use of nitrites in meats', *Food Technology*, 34 (1980), pp. 254–57.

97. 'Plan to ban nitrites in foods dropped for now', *Chemical and Engineering News*, 25 August 1980, p. 11.

98. *New Scientist*, 24 August 1978, p. 35.

99. Miller, 'Balancing the risks'.

100. Lois R. Ember, 'Nitrosamines – assessing the relative risk', *Chemical and Engineering News*, 31 March 1980, pp. 20–26.

101. *Ibid*.

102. *Ibid*.

103. Figures issued by Family Planning Association in 1978.

104. O. Gillie, *Sunday Times*, 24 September 1978.

105. L. J. Kinlen *et al*., 'A survey of the use of oestrogens during pregnancy in the UK and of the genito-urinary cancer mortality

and incidence rates in young people in England and Wales', *Journal of Obstetrics and Gynaecology of the British Commonwealth*, 81 (1974), pp. 849–55.

106. J. W. Murray, 'Hormone scare knocks the European veal market', *Observer*, 28 September 1980.

107. 'World report', *Observer*, 21 September 1980.

108. A. L. Herbst, H. Ulfelder, D. C. Poskanzer, 'Adenocarcinoma of the vagina: association of maternal stilbestrol therapy with tumor appearance in young women', *New England Journal of Medicine*, 284 (1971), pp. 878–81.

109. See, for example, A. L. Herbst *et al.*, 'Clear-cell adenocarcinoma of the genital tract in young females', *New England Journal of Medicine*, 287 (1972), p. 1259.

110. See, for example, A. Stafl and R. F. Mattingly, 'Vaginal adenosis: a precancerous lesion?', *American Journal of Obstetrics and Gynecology*, vol. 120, no. 5 (1974), pp. 666–77.

111. R. H. Kaufman *et al.*, 'Upper genital tract changes associated with exposure in utero to diethylstilbestrol', *American Journal of Obstetrics and Gynecology*, 128 (1977), pp. 51–59.

112. A. B. Barnes *et al.*, 'Fertility and outcome of pregnancy in women exposed in utero to diethylstilbestrol', *New England Journal of Medicine*, 302 (1980), pp. 609–13.

113. M. D. Cosgrove, B. Benton and B. E. Henderson, 'Male genito-urinary abnormalities and maternal diethylstilbestrol', *Journal of Urology*, 117 (1977), pp. 220–22.

114. M. Bibbo *et al.*, 'A 25-year follow-up study of women exposed to diethylstilbestrol during pregnancy', *New England Journal of Medicine*, 298 (1978), pp. 763–67.

115. W. J. Dieckmann *et al.*, 'Does the administration of diethylstil-bestrol during pregnancy have therapeutic value?', *American Journal of Obstetrics and Gynecology*, 66 (1953), pp. 1062–81. For an account of how pregnant women were persuaded to take DES in a major USA hospital see S. Epstein, *The Politics of Cancer*, pp. 224–26.

116. Y. Brackbill and H. W. Berendes, 'Dangers of diethylstilbestrol: a review of a 1953 paper', *Lancet*, 2 (1978), p. 520.

117. F. M. Sullivan, 'The teratogenic and other toxic effects of drugs on reproduction', in P. F. D'Arcy and J. P. Griffin (eds), *Iatrogenic Diseases*, Oxford University Press (2nd edn, 1979).

118. WHO Scientific Group Report, *The Effect of Female Sex Hormones on Fetal Development and Infant Health*, World Health Organisation (1981).

119. S. Silverberg *et al.*, 'Endometrial carcinoma in women under 40 years of age: comparison of cases in oral contraceptive users and non-users', *Cancer*, 39 (1977), pp. 592–98.

120. International Agency for Research on Cancer, *Evaluation of the Carcinogenic Risk of Chemicals to Man. Vol. 6 Sex Hormones*, Lyon, France (1974).

121. J. Neuberger, 'Oral contraceptive-associated liver tumours: occurrence of malignancy and difficulties in diagnosis', *Lancet*, 1 (1980), pp. 273–76.

122. M. Vessey *et al.*, 'A long-term follow-up study of women using different methods of contraception: a interim report', *Journal of Biosocial Science*, 8 (1976), pp. 373–427.

123. E. Stern, 'Contraceptives and dysplasia: higher rate for pill-choosers', *Science*, 196 (1977), pp. 1,460–62.

124. J. Rakusen, 'Depo-Provera: the extent of the problem – a case study in the politics of birth control', in H. Roberts (ed.), *Women, Health and Reproduction*, Routledge & Kegan Paul (1981).

125. Family Planning Information Service, *Fact Sheet*, no. 31, May 1979.

126. 'Depo-Provera may be linked to uterine cancer, preliminary data imply', *Family Planning Perspectives*, 11 (1979), p. 47.

127. *Times*, 30 April 1982.

128. M. Fathy and E. I. Etreby, 'Effect of contraceptive steroids on mammary tumour development in experimental animals', *Trends in Pharmacological Science*, 1 (1980), pp. 362–65.

129. S. Epstein, *The Politics of Cancer*, pp. 221–22.

130. M. I. Whitehead *et al.*, 'Progestogen modification of estrogen-induced endometrial proliferation in climacteric women', in I. D. Cooke (ed.), *The Role of Estrogen/Progestogen in the Management of the Menopause*, MIT Press, Massachusetts (1978).

131. C. M. F. Antunes *et al.*, 'Endometrial cancer and estrogen use: report of a large case control study', *New England Journal of Medicine*, 300 (1979), pp. 9–13.

132. H. Jick *et al.*, 'Replacement estrogens and endometrial cancer', *New England Journal of Medicine*, 300 (1979), pp. 218–22.

133. B. Howard, *Daily Telegraph*, 31 January 1980.

6. Case studies: the general environment

1. For details of the evidence of the carcinogenicity of A/D and C/H see S. Epstein, *The Politics of Cancer*, Anchor Press (1979), chapter 7.

2. For details, see *ibid.*, pp. 256–58.

3. *Ibid.*, p. 270.

4. K. W. Jager, *Aldrin, Dieldrin, Endrin and Telodrin*, Elsevier, Amsterdam (1970).

5. Quoted in B. Gillespie, 'British control of pesticide technology', unpublished PhD thesis, University of Manchester (1977).

6. *British Medical Journal*, 25 January 1975, p. 170; *Lancet*, 2 (1974), p. 629; *Lancet*, 1 (1976), p. 571.

7. Epstein, *The Politics of Cancer*, chapter 7.

8. See J. Matthews, 'Unions press for herbicide ban', *New Scientist*, 12 February 1980, pp. 558–60.

9. S. Epstein, Testimony on Agent Orange and HR 1961, House Committee on Veterans' Affairs, US Congress, 27 April 1983; for a detailed discussion of the chemistry of 2,4,5-T as well as its history see A. Hay, *The Chemical Scythe: Lessons of 2,4,5-T and Dioxin*, Plenum, 1982.

10. Hay, *The Chemical Scythe*, chapter 7.

11. O. Axelson *et al.*, 'Herbicide exposure and tumor mortality: an updated epidemiological investigation of Swedish railroad workers', *Lakartidningen*, 76 (1979) p. 3505; L. Hardell and A. Sandstrom, 'Case control study: soft tissue sarcomas and exposure to phenoxyacetic acids or chlorophenols', *British Journal of Cancer*, 39 (1979), pp. 711–17; Ton That Tung, 'Le cancer primaire du foie au Viet-nam', *Chirurgie*, 99 (1973), pp. 427–36; R. Cook, 'Dioxin, chloracne and soft tissue sarcoma, *Lancet* (1981), pp. 618–19.

12. Hay, *The Chemical Scythe*, Chapter 7.

13. See chapter 3 for further discussion of the regulatory structure.

14. NUAAW, *Not One Minute Longer*, reprinted July 1980.

15. *Ibid.*, p. 3.

16. R. Thomas, G. Wardell and D. Williams, '2,4,5-T cover-up by the MAFF', *Ecologist*, vol. 10, nos 6/7 (1980), pp. 249–51.

17. The resolution was proposed by the NUAAW.

18. MAFF, Advisory Committee on Pesticides, *Further Review of the Safety for Use in the UK of the Herbicide, 2,4,5-T*, HMSO (1980). A further report was produced by a subcommittee of the ACP in early 1983 where again 2,4,5-T was given a clean bill of health.

19. J. Cook and C. Kaufman, *Portrait of a Poison*, Pluto Press (1982).

7. How industry resists regulation

1. T. Kletz, 'What risks should we run?', in *The Risk Equations,* New Scientist (1978).

2. J. Cook and C. Kaufman, *Portrait of a Poison*, Pluto Press (1982).

3. A. W. Barnes, 'National and International Aspects of the VC Health Problem', BPF/PRI Joint Conference (May 1975), p. 13.
4. Chemical Industries Association, *The Control of Occupational Cancer*, CIA Position Paper (November 1981).
5. C. Clutterbuck, 'Death in the plastics factory', *Radical Science Journal*, 4 (1976).
6. 'Clean up cover up', *Hazards Bulletin*, 18 (1980).
7. ASTMS, *The Prevention of Occupational Cancer – An ASTMS Policy Document* (February 1980).
8. J. Keir Howard, *'The Prevention of Occupational Cancer – An ASTMS Policy Document: a review'*, CIA Background Paper (June 1980).
9. *Cancer in Modern Mortality*, CIA Publications (1980).
10. Chemical Industries Association, *Control of Occupational Cancer*, 1981.
11. GMWU/ASTMS, *Response to CIA Paper on Occupational Carcinogens* (June 1982).
12. A. Dalton, *Asbestos: Killer Dust*, BSSRS (1979), pp. 59–60.
13. 'CISHEC – the Chemical Industry Safety and Health Council', CIA Publications (undated), p. 4.
14. 'Genetic association with bladder cancer', *British Medical Journal* (September 1979), p. 514.
15. S. Epstein, *The Politics of Cancer*, Anchor Press, New York (1979), p. 432; J. Ives, *The Export of Hazardous Industries*, Praeger, New York (1981); M. Dowie *et al.*, 'The Corporate Crime of the Century', *Mother Jones*, November 1979.
16. 'Banned chemical produced', *Hazards Bulletin*, 17 (1979).
17. A. Dalton, *Asbestos: Killer Dust*, p. 244.
18. 'Kenyan farmers risk their lives for smokers', *New Scientist*, 8 April 1982, p. 67. See also D. Bull, *A Growing Problem: Pesticides and the Third World Poor*, Oxfam (1982).
19. M. Muller, *Tobacco and the Third World: Tomorrow's Epidemic?*, War on Want (1978).
20. 'Further nonsense on product liability', *Nature*, 1288 (1980), p. 526.
21. N. A. Ashford, G. R. Heaton and W. C. Priest, 'Environmental, health and safety regulations and technological innovation', in C. T. Hill and G. M. Utterback (eds), *Technological Innovation in a Dynamic Economy*, Pergamon (1979).
22. N. A. Ashford and G. R. Heaton, 'Government regulation: the impact on technological innovation', *Professional Engineer*, vol. 45, no. 12 (1975), pp. 31–33. Our emphasis.
23. This is one of several examples of net savings from health, safety and

environmental controls quoted in R. Kazis and R. L. Grossman, *Fear at Work: Job Blackmail, Labour and the Environment*, Pilgrim Press (1982). See also S. Epstein, L. O. Brown and C. Pope, *Hazardous Waste in America*, Sierra Club Books, San Francisco (1982), chapters 12 and 13.

24. *Health, Safety and The Environment*, Chemicals EDC Discussion Document (1981).

8. How to fight back: the politics of prevention

1. Alliance for Safety and Health, *Toxic Ireland*, Dublin (1982). See also S. Epstein, L. O. Brown and C. Pope, *Hazardous Waste in America*, Sierra Club Books, San Francisco (1982).

2. A. Dalton, *Asbestos: Killer Dust*, BSSRS (1979).

3. A good one is P. Parish, *Medicines: A Guide for Everybody*, Penguin, Harmondsworth (1977).

4. If you need help, you could also read the chapter on birth control in Boston Women's Health Book Collective, *Our Bodies Ourselves*, British edition by Angela Phillips and Jill Rakusen, Penguin, Harmondsworth (1980).

5. For a detailed list of these products see J. Cook and C. Kaufman, *Portrait of a Poison*, Pluto Press (1982).

6. CIA, *The Control of Occupational Carcinogens: A CIA Position Paper* (November 1981), p. 3.

7. Science Council of Canada, *Policies and Poisons – The Containment of Long-Term Hazards to Human Health in the Environment and the Workplace*, (October 1977).

8. L. Doyal, 'A matter of life and death', in J. Irvine, I. Miles and J. Evans (eds), *Demystifying Social Statistics*, Pluto Press (1979); Radical Statistics Health Group, *The Unofficial Guide to Official Health Statistics* (1980), available from BSSRS, 9 Poland Street, London W1V 3DG.

9. J. Michael, *The Politics of Secrecy: The Case for a Freedom of Information Law*, National Council for Civil Liberties (1979); Freedom of Information Campaign, *Secrecy, or the Right to Know?*, Library Association (1980); T. Barnes, *Open Up: Britain and Freedom of Information in the 1980s*, Fabian Tract 467 (1980); R. Delbridge and M. Smith (eds), *Consuming Secrets: How Official Secrecy Affects Everyday Life in Britain*, Burnett Books (1982).

10. R. Macrory and B. Zaba, *The Control of Pollution Act Explained*, Friends of the Earth (1978). See also M. Frankel in R. Delbridge and A. Smith (eds), *Consuming Secrets*.

11. *Guardian*, 28 January 1977.
12. Michael, *The Politics of Secrecy*, p. 13.
13. M. Peters, 'Lead in petrol: the politics of the science of lead pollution', *Radical Science Journal*, 10 (1980), pp. 102–7.

Index

Lesley Doyal (with Imogen Pennell)
The Political Economy of Health

'It marks the turning point in the study of health, illness and health care which brings together for the first time much collective thinking by the health workers, feminists, sociologists and economists on both sides of the Atlantic and in the Third World.' *Marxism Today*

'This is a cut above the usual polemical book on health and health services. It is readable and well researched... Altogether a stimulating book and a worthy contribution to current debates on the politics of health' *The Lancet*

'Mandatory reading for anyone with the slightest interest in health — including doctors.' *New Statesman*

0 86104 074 0   paperback   £4.95

Bobbie Jacobson

The Ladykillers

why smoking is a feminist issue (including a guide to
giving up)

The Ladykillers should be required reading' *Women in Medicine*

'the only available study on the subject... comprehensive and succinct
volume' *Sunday Times*

'an excellent feminist book on women and smoking. In it she
explores why women smoke and offers some interesting and
supportive suggestions for a women's strategy for quitting' *Spare Rib*

0 86104 341 3   paperback   £2.50

Colin Thunhurst
It Makes You Sick
the politics of the NHS

Today the National Health Service is on the point of collapse and private health care schemes are burgeoning. Colin Thunhurst shows how the potential of the NHS has been undermined by successive governments ever since its inception. He argues that this is a product of the society we live in — that modern capitalism creates ill-health and profits from it.

It Makes You Sick proposes policies for re-shaping and democratising the NHS in order to make it a genuinely egalitarian system of health care.

'**It Makes You Sick** is an excellent and balanced introduction to the organisation and problems of the health services, while making clear the economic and social basis of much ill-health' *Tribune*

'written with force, lucidity and precision' *New Statesman*

0 86104 503 3   paperback   £2.50

Vicente Navarro (Editor)
Imperialism, Health and Medicine

The essays in this collection examine various aspects of what has
been called the 'underdevelopment of health'. They reject the widely-
held view that poverty and ill-health are caused by over-population,
arguing instead that they have to be seen as part of the human
destruction wrought by capitalist expansion throughout the world.
Issues explored include: the politics of food aid; the ideological
influence of western medicine in the third world; the export of
hazardous industries and unhealthy commodities to underdeveloped
countries, and the political economy of population control.

'The themes under review here are profoundly disturbing and
crucially important... a book to be read.' *The Health Services*

0 86104 375 8   paperback   £6.95

Pluto books are available through your local bookshop. In case of
difficulty contact Pluto to find out local stocklists or to obtain
catalogues/leaflets. If all else fails write to:

Pluto Press Limited
Freepost, (no stamp required)
105A, Torriano Avenue
London NW5 1YP

To order, enclose a cheque/p.o. payable to Pluto Press to cover price
of book, plus 50p per book for postage and packing
(£2.50 maximum). Telephone 01-482 1973.